Understanding Health Care Outcomes Research

Edited by

Robert L. Kane, MD

Professor and Director
Clinical Outcomes Research Center
University of Minnesota
Minneapolis, Minnesota

JONES AND BARTLETT PUBLISHERS
Sudbury, Massachusetts

BOSTON   TORONTO   LONDON   SINGAPORE

World Headquarters
Jones and Bartlett Publishers
40 Tall Pine Drive
Sudbury, MA 01776
978-443-5000
info@jbpub.com
www.jbpub.com

Jones and Bartlett Publishers Canada
2406 Nikanna Road
Mississauga, ON L5C 2W6
CANADA

Jones and Bartlett Publishers International
Barb House, Barb Mews
London W6 7PA
UK

ISBN 0-7637- 2628-1

Production Credits
Publisher: Michael Brown
Production Manager: Amy Rose
Associate Production Editor: Karen C. Ferreira
Marketing Manager: Joy Stark-Vancs
Manufacturing Buyer: Amy Bacus
Printing and Binding: RR Donnelley
Cover Printing: RR Donnelley

Printed in the United States of America
08 07 06 05 04   10 9 8 7 6 5 4 3 2 1

Table of Contents_____

Foreword

Outcomes information, whether used for research or within the context of clinical practice, holds the promise of bridging the gap between what is done and what the intervention actually accomplishes. Health services research has contributed greatly to the understanding of effectiveness by bringing the patient perspective into the forefront. The use of patient self-reported health and functional status measures, in addition to clinical outcomes, is changing the way research is conducted and medicine is practiced.

Health care systems constantly struggle with ways to provide higher quality care in a cost-effective manner. Risk-sharing arrangements are moving health care systems into a model of improving health, as well as treating illness. For example, managed care groups are looking for ways to encourage people toward "wellness" in the form of healthier lifestyles and work environments. Administrators of managed care systems know that the only way to truly reduce the cost of health care and increase their success is to improve the health of their members, decrease utilization, and increase the likelihood of appropriate care. Concurrently, the consumers of health care are demanding changes in the way health is viewed. The emerging definition is one where health is defined, not as the absence of disease, but as the ability to function fully–physically, emotionally, socially, and spiritually–within the context of the lives we construct and the expectations we set.

Measuring outcomes is a first step in the assessment of the patient perspective and in determining the consequence of health care. Outcomes research is providing the groundwork necessary to enable effective clinical decisions that relate to the context and quality of life. Moving the use of outcomes data into the course of clinical care increases the likelihood that medical care will improve the health, functional status, and well-being of patients.

This book provides a welcome and much-needed introduction to the utility of outcomes data in the process of making clinical decisions. Dr. Kane and all of the contributors to this book provide a straightforward and demystifying view of outcomes research. *Understanding Health Care Outcomes Research* contributes an eloquent voice in the reasoning of why this type of research is important and valid.

I believe this book will become a requisite resource to health services researchers and clinicians who utilize patient-centered outcomes information in the context of care. My hope is that it promotes further work in the evolution of a patient-centered approach to clinical decision making, and helps to bridge the gap between the treatment of illness and a return to health and functionality.

– Ellen B. White
President and Chief Executive Officer
Velocity Healthcare Informatics, Inc.
Minneapolis, Minnesota

Preface

Interest in studying the outcomes of care is increasing rapidly for several reasons. The demand for accountability has fostered new emphasis on examining what happens to patients. Closely linked to accountability is the increased use of quality improvement techniques, usually associated with movements from the manufacturing sector, such as continuous quality improvement and total quality management.

Much of the press for improving quality relies heavily on examining and correcting the process of care. Methods for ensuring the appropriateness of care, such as the use of clinical protocols (or their less threatening counterpart, guidelines) often are used. The enthusiasm for guidelines presupposes that solid information exists to identify the appropriate way to provide care for designated patients. Such information must be derived from solid evidence of the link between what is done and the effects of this action. In short, appropriateness requires proof of effectiveness.

Some have urged that attention be directed to proving effectiveness before advocating standards for effectiveness. Efforts to establish the effectiveness of care require careful study of how treatment affects outcomes. Some of this evidence can come from experimental studies, but most will have to come from carefully performed observational analyses and quasi-experimental studies, using tactics derived from epidemiology. Many approach such studies with great trepidation because they fear they can never point a causal arrow directly from treatment to outcomes; too many other factors can confound the picture.

Outcomes research differs from more traditional clinical research largely in its attention to a wider range of outcomes. Whereas the traditional measures of treatment success used in clinical research (such as preventing or delaying death and improving specific physiologic parameters) can still apply, outcomes research pays more attention to patient-centered outcomes. These may include measures of physical function, such as the ability to perform various tasks; they may address an overall sense of improved well-being; or they may cover a wider range of measures that have been termed *health-related quality of life*. In many instances, the concern about outcomes has been couched in terms of cost-effectiveness– essentially, what improvement in health status is generated for a given level of resources? Or, how much "bang" is obtained for the "buck"?

In the new generation of health research, recognizing the importance of patient-centered outcome measures has become *de rigueur*. Many clinical trials now include a broad outcome measure to cover this aspect. Too often the measure is selected for its brevity as much as for its value. When most clinicians think about outcomes, they are hoping for some simple summary measures that can encompass all of human suffering in a single statistic. This naive search for the holy grail of outcomes reflects an underlying failure to grasp the real intent of such measures. The outcomes of care are multifaceted and complex. Measurement cannot simplify what is essentially complicated. No single index can adequately portray the vicissitudes of life.

This book is intended to assist those who have been assigned the task (or who have sought the opportunity) to develop outcomes studies for their organizations or for investigators who want to undertake such studies to pursue knowledge about what works in medical care. It is designed to reassure on the one hand and stimulate on the other. The reassurance comes by providing new investigators with insights to help them undertake this work with an awareness of what is needed to conduct successful studies. Although there is clearly a value in experimental studies, such as randomized clinical trials, much useful information can be gleaned from well-done quasiexperimental studies. In both cases, careful planning, based on a clear conceptual model of the expected relationships among the variables of interest, is necessary. Outcomes research is not simply about developing mathematical models to explain observed phenomena. It is intended to explore causal pathways. In many cases, it will require sophisticated analytic methods to try to compensate for potential variation in what cannot be controlled. Its results should be presented thoughtfully and modestly but without apology. The authors of this book hope it will stimulate new insights by allowing more established investigators to appreciate some of the subtle and not-so-subtle aspects of outcomes research.

For those embarking on this journey as relative neophytes, we offer the following principles:

1. Outcomes research is feasible. It must be done carefully, but it can yield useful information.
2. Conducting solid outcomes research requires careful attention to basic design and to the subtleties of each situation. One must begin with a clear question and not hope that the analysis will yield spontaneous insight.

3. A careful delineation of the factors that might influence the outcomes of interest and a conceptual model of the expected relationships among those factors are essential.
4. Technical issues are important. Aspects of measurement theory apply. Appropriate statistical analysis, often using sophisticated methods to correct for such problems as potential selection bias, is needed. Consultation in advance with statisticians and methodologists is strongly recommended.

The authors hope that this book will prove useful as a source of inspiration and insight. It is designed less as a step-by-step how-to-do-it manual than a treatise on the important issues that surround outcomes research.

– Robert L. Kane, M.D.
Editor

1

Approaching the Outcomes Question

Robert L. Kane

CHAPTER OUTLINE

- What Types of Study Designs Can Be Used in Outcomes Research?
- What Is an Outcomes Approach?
- What is Risk Adjustment?
- What Does Treatment Include for Outcomes Researchers?
- How Are Outcomes Measured?
- What Is the First Step?
- How Is This Book Organized?

Outcomes of care have suddenly become big news. Like Moliere's bourgeois gentilhomme who suddenly discovered he had been speaking prose all his life, health care providers seem to have awakened to the need to examine the results of their labors. It is not totally clear what precipitated this revolution. A combination of factors seems to be responsible. Especially at a time when health care costs are skyrocketing, the observations about the large variation in the rates of various medical activities and utilization of care stirred interest in whether these differences had any effect on outcomes. The rise of managed care, with its industrial accountability and productivity models, stimulated a revised way of thinking about care. As the variation data generated a press for greater consistency, which was translated into a demand for clinical guidelines, it became quickly evident that medicine does not have a vast store of empirically verified information about the relationship between what is done and the results.

Outcomes analysis can be undertaken for several reasons:

- **To make market decisions.** In an ideal world, consumers looking for help might want to know how well a given clinician has performed in treating their specific problem. Likewise, those acting on behalf of consumers (e.g., benefits managers) might want such information to help in their decisions about with whom to contract.

- **To provide accountability.** Several agencies have a stake in the quality of medical care. Formal regulatory activity is vested in the government and in professional societies. Payers may also be concerned that the care they are buying is of adequate quality. In effect, the same information on the outcomes achieved can be analyzed at the level of a clinician, or a clinic, or a hospital (if the sample size is large enough). In conducting such analyses, however, appropriate adjustments for case mix and other relevant risk factors are needed in both cases.

- **To improve the knowledge base of medicine.** The enthusiasm for establishing guidelines for care has been somewhat dampened by the growing realization that the empirical database for most of these recommendations is quite weak, and this fact forces a reliance on clinical consensus judgments. While some would hold that the only real science comes from randomized controlled trials (RCT), much can be learned by carefully applying epidemiological analyses to large databases of well-collected experiential information.

Outcomes can be expressed in different ways. Clinicians are most familiar with clinical measures ranging from death to values of specific parameters like blood pressure. Outcomes also can be derived from symptoms or even the results of physical examinations. They can be the results of simple tests, like blood levels, or more complex physiological measures. Another set of outcomes relies on information collected from patients. Such data usually reflect how patients have experienced the illness and the effects it has had on their lives. These outcomes include measures of functioning as well as measures of affect. Satisfaction with care and with life in general can be considered part of this set of outcomes. In general, clinicians place greater faith in the data they get from laboratory tests and their own observations than what patients report, but this prejudice may not be appropriate. Patient-derived information can be as valid as, or even more valid than, that obtained from a machine. For example, the results of a scale based on patient perceptions of events may be as valid as the inference placed on the results of a colorimetric reaction that is interpreted as reflecting the level of enzymatic activity.

Looking directly at the outcomes of care (as opposed to concentrating on the process of care) makes a lot of sense. In the best traditions of Willie Sutton (who said he robbed banks because that was where the money was), outcomes are where the treasure can be found. However, using outcomes may be less satisfying than one may wish. Clinicians have difficulties with outcomes on several grounds:

- **The outcomes of care may be due to many things, only some of which are under the clinician's control.** It is much more satisfying to be able to say you did all the right things, even if something bad happened. Some estimates suggest that medical care has only a limited effect on the overall health of a population. It seems reasonable to assume that the size of the effect of treatment on specific sick people is larger, but other factors will still influence the results. It is not necessary that treatment explain all (or even most) of the variance on outcomes to make it worthwhile to examine its effectiveness. One can change the risk of a successful outcome by several orders of magnitude by interventions that fail to explain even a modest amount of the variance in outcomes.

- **Although theory suggests that outcomes and process measures are closely linked, a poor outcome does not immediately suggest what needs to be done differently.** At best, outcomes can only tell an investigator where to look for more information. In clinical practice, they are best thought of as screeners. Rather than examining the processes of care for all the care provided, a pattern of poor outcomes can suggest which types of care (or which providers) need closer scrutiny.

- **Outcomes information usually requires extra effort (and expense) to collect.** Medical practice does not routinely gather systematic information about the outcomes of care. At best, clinicians are generally aware of only those patients who return for further care. Rarely do they systematically follow the course of their care. Even less often do they collect data on other variables that might influence the outcomes.

- **Outcomes are essentially probability statements.** Because outcomes can be influenced by many different factors, one should not try to judge the success of any single case. Rather, outcomes are addressed in the aggregate. The rate of success is compared. Thus, outcomes reflect the experience of a clinician, not the results of any single effort.

- **Outcome results take a long time to assemble.** First, one must accumulate cases. For each case, one must wait for the outcomes to become evident.

- **In some cases, the ultimate outcome may lie far off in the future, and some sort of intermediate outcome must be used.** For example, control of blood sugar in diabetes may serve as a proxy outcome for the real goal of preventing complications such as limb or vision loss.

Given all these problems, it is little wonder that people would rather talk about outcomes than deal with them. It is much more comfortable to test the extent to which care complies with extant orthodoxy. However, one quickly runs into a paradox. Clinicians too often base their decisions about what constitutes appropriate care on beliefs rather than hard evidence. Before an orthodoxy is endorsed, there should be better proof that a given approach really leads to better outcomes. Developing such linkages means having a data system that can provide the needed grist for the analytic mill.

Two strategies are available to collect outcomes information:

1. Routine medical practice can incorporate system data collection and feedback to track outcomes of care. The rise of managed care, with its improved information systems and its concerns about efficiency, may prove a catalyst for this effort.
2. Certain practice sites can be designated (under a special franchise arrangement) to operate data-collection activities under some scientific aegis that would systematically collect data on outcomes and relate them to the process of care (much the way academic centers conduct clinical trials to test new therapies). Practitioners would then rely on the validated processes for assessing their quality of care.

Having recognized the discrepancy between what is known and what is believed, medicine was at an impasse. One camp, anxious for fast results, pushed for creating practice guidelines based on the best available information and filling in the rest with expert opinion. They argued that, at worst, such a strategy would produce the equivalent of a higher quality textbook. The other camp maintained that enforcing arbitrary rules not based on empirical evidence is equivalent to codifying beliefs. They urged greater restraint until a better science base was developed.

The early experience with guideline writing confirmed the weak science base that underlies much of clinical practice. The big question is how to remedy the situation. Systematic outcomes research is the obvious answer. The choice of the best research strategy remains the question.

The classical view of quality of medical care uses a framework that divides such work into structure, process, and outcome (Donabedian, 1966). *Structure* refers to such aspects as the training of the care providers or the equipment of the facility in which the care is provided. *Process* addresses what was done: Was the correct (appropriate) action taken? Was it done skillfully? *Outcomes* refers to the results of these actions. There is an assumption that these three aspects are directly related, but that belief has often proven hard to demonstrate empirically. One explanation is that the "lore" of medicine is just that, a set of beliefs and traditions that are poorly grounded in empirical evidence. Another interpretation is that the effects of care are simply too subtle to be easily revealed by most studies, especially nonexperimental ones.

The weak relationships often found between process and structure on the one hand and outcomes on the other cut both ways. Investigators seeking to demonstrate the validity of their outcomes findings may turn to structural and process correlations. If outcome measures work, one would expect to find better outcomes among those providers judged by some external standard to give better care. What does it mean when care provided in teaching hospitals is no better than that offered in community hospitals? On the one hand, the measures may be insensitive; alternatively, there may be less difference than one suspects. If the results are the inverse of what is expected, there will obviously be greater cause for concern, but failure to find a difference where orthodox teaching says one should be found may raise at least as many questions about the orthodoxy as challenges to the validity of the observation.

WHAT TYPES OF STUDY DESIGNS CAN BE USED IN OUTCOMES RESEARCH?

Clinical research worships at the shrine of the RCT. The ability to assign subjects randomly to either experimental or control status confers an aura of science that is unsurpassed.[1] Indeed, serious questions of bias can arise whenever the decision to treat or not (or how to treat) is determined by some external force. Those reviewing the results of nonrandomized studies need to be reassured that potential risk factors have been identified and addressed. Nonetheless, there remains a concern that the experimental and control groups are not completely comparable and, hence, that unknown factors may account for differences found. A number of statistical procedures have been developed to address this issue, but the level of comfort with the results of these efforts varies with the discipline. Clinicians, who are usually not statistically sophisticated, need a lot of reassurance that the experimental and control groups are comparable.

In general, randomized trials use great care in design to specify inclusion criteria. Because RCTs are complicated and difficult to mount, they are usually restricted to very tightly targeted groups of patients. Often, the investigators are not actively concerned about how the subjects are obtained and rely on random allocation to distribute any differences equally across the two groups. As a result, randomized trials often trade internal validity (tightness of comparisons) for external validity (generalizability). Thus, randomization does not provide the protective shield that some think. Even if the groups are more comparable (and such a distribution is not ensured by random assignment), the pertinent analyses may still require looking at the data within subclasses. It does not seem feasible to rely exclusively on RCTs for all, or even most, of the needed empirical data linking outcomes to the process of care.

There are those who maintain that nothing but RCTs can provide real evidence of efficacy. Epidemiological models applied to observational data can never be absolutely sure that differences found were not due to unobserved variations in the two groups. Random allocation is a powerful tool, but both because of other limitations (especially in regard to examining the effectiveness of a treatment, i.e., how it actually works in practice) and simply for reasons of logistics, epidemiological studies will inevitably play a major role.

In effect, both approaches require some level of extrapolation and inference. The RCT requires a heavy set of inferences to extrapolate the results based on extensive participant selection and fixed interventions to clinical practice. The epidemiological approach requires a substantial amount of inference in the analysis itself, but the translation to practice is thus much easier because many of the relevant variables have already been addressed.

Because the epidemiological approach is essentially a naturalistic technique that relies on data collected as part of extant practice, questions will arise about the comparability of those who receive different forms of care. The assignment to treatment groups is not based on chance. Factors, both overt and more subtle, determine who gets what care. The burden of proof lies with the investigator. In truth, no amount of evidence can absolutely guarantee comparability, but a lot of informational benefit can accrue from using carefully analyzed information derived from real practice.

A much more important problem in using clinical information is its quality. Clinical investigators quickly appreciate that clinical data are not recorded systematically or thoroughly. Patient information is entered when patients visit the system. No systematic follow-up is obtained. Much of the information recorded summarizes clinicians' overall impressions rather than capturing the presence of specific signs and symptoms. Two clinicians may opt to record quite disparate information, even when they use the same headings. The meaning of clinical terms may vary from one clinician to another. In some cases, the same term means different things; in others, different terms mean the same thing. Investigators seeking to mount outcomes studies will need to plan these studies to include prospective data collection and incorporate deliberate steps that attend to the quality of information at each stage.

WHAT IS AN OUTCOMES APPROACH?

An outcomes approach requires more than simply collecting data on the outcomes of care. It should be thought of in terms of an outcomes information system. Careful and complete data collection for purposes of both outcomes ascertainment and risk adjustment has to be combined with proper analyses.

The basic model for analyzing the outcomes of care is the same whether one uses an RCT or an epidemiological approach. The model can be summarized as follows:

Outcomes = f(baseline, patient clinical characteristics, patient demographic/psychosocial characteristics, treatment, setting)

This formula indicates that clinical outcomes are the result of several factors, which can be classified as risk factors (baseline status, clinical status, and demographic/psychosocial characteristics) and treatment characteristics (treatment and setting).[2] The goal of the analysis is to isolate the relationship between the outcomes of interest and the treatment provided by controlling for the effects of other relevant material. The latter is often referred to as *risk adjustment.*

WHAT IS RISK ADJUSTMENT?

Essentially, risk adjustment is an effort to create a level playing field. Every physician seems to believe that he or she cares for the toughest cases. Comparisons of outcomes among practitioners, hospitals, or any other way of comparing providers must attempt to correct adequately for the differences in the composition of the patients who are being treated by each. The salient risk factors can include patients' demographic descriptors, their clinical characteristics, and their status at the time they present for treatment (and even their usual health status before they became ill).

The patient's baseline status is very important. With a few exceptions (such as plastic surgery and elective orthopaedics), most medical treatment does not get a patient better than he or she was before the episode that started the need for treatment in the first place. Thus, there are really two types of baseline status information that need to be collected: (1) status at the outset of treatment (which can be used to show how much change has occurred since treatment began) and (2) usual status before the onset of the problem that requires treatment (which defines the upper bound of just how much improvement is possible or likely). Information on baseline status basically corresponds to what will be collected later to assess outcomes.

Patient clinical characteristics cover a lot of territory. One of the reasons clinicians make diagnoses is to group patients into classes that share a need for a given type of therapy and/or to suggest an expected course. Knowing a patient's diagnosis would thus play a central role in building an outcomes data system. Many patients have more than one diagnosis. It is necessary for purposes of analysis to identify one diagnosis as the primary diagnosis and to treat the others as modifiers.[3] These are often referred to as *comorbidities.*

Diagnoses can be further refined in terms of their implications for outcomes by addressing characteristics that suggest varying prognoses. These are termed *severity measures*. In addition to severity, one may be concerned about other modifiers of diagnoses, such as duration of the problem and history of previous episodes. In general, it is usually safer to be as inclusive as possible. Because clinicians are especially distrustful of non-RCTs, they need a great deal of reassurance that all possible differences between groups have been considered. By bending over to include elements that seem unnecessary, the investigator may eventually gain greater acceptance for the results. Nothing is more frustrating than presenting an analysis, especially one that challenges conventional wisdom, only to have the clinical audience say: "Yes, but did you consider . . .?" A policy of inclusion is not an automatic talisman against rejection, but it can help avoid it. At some point, of course, the cost of collecting seemingly irrelevant data can be overwhelming. A reasonable compromise must be struck. If the clinician audience is involved in planning the study, at least those elements that seem most important can be covered. Other clinical information may address different risk factors (e.g., exposure to toxins, diet, or habits).

The other set of patient information concerns demographic and psychosocial factors. Some obvious items like age and gender seem to need no justification, but even they should be thoughtfully addressed. A specific conceptual model that indicates the expected influence of each variable is a critical first step in planning an outcomes study. Others, such as education and social support, may exert their effects more subtly. The relevance of specific elements may vary with the condition being examined. Other psychosocial variables, including the patient's cognitive or emotional state, may influence the effects of treatment on other outcomes.

WHAT DOES TREATMENT INCLUDE FOR OUTCOMES RESEARCHERS?

Setting refers to both the physical location where the care is provided as well as the organization of that site. It can also address other attributes, such as the philosophy of care provided. For example, one may want to compare the same basic care provided in an inpatient and outpatient context. Alternatively, one may want to address the level of risk aversion or the extent of staffing for apparently similar models of care. One site may have a philosophy of encouraging patients to do as much as possible for themselves; another may be inclined to provide a lot of services to assist patients in performing basic activities, either because they are concerned about safety or because they feel that doing things for patients may be faster in the long run.

At its most basic level, *treatment* can refer simply to gross types; for example, does medical management work better than surgical? It can even be simply a proxy for care given in one hospital versus another or by one physician versus others. Measuring the effects of treatment first requires a clear, useful taxonomy for treatments. Surprisingly little work has gone into creating such schema. Just as one needs to think not only about formal treatments like prescribed drugs but also about over-the-counter medications, the definition of a therapy may not be limited to what is done in a clinical setting. Informal care may play a substantial role. In some cases, the treatment may extend over several sites. For example, much of the care formerly rendered in hospitals is now provided in nursing homes and even at home.

A simple model to classify treatment can be derived from drug therapy, where one talks about such constructs as type, dosage, duration, and timing. A similar approach can be taken to other treatments, such as surgery. The next level of analysis might ask whether the same treatment in different hands produces different results. At this point, the issue becomes individual skill.

Treatment relates directly to Donabedian's (1966) process of care, which can be said to be composed of two basic aspects: (1) doing the right/appropriate thing and (2) doing it well. The goal of outcomes research is to establish what treatment is appropriate for a given situation by isolating the effects of treatment from the effects of other factors that influence outcomes. It is harder to use outcomes to address skill than to establish appropriateness. Typically, skill is assessed by direct observation. Another clinician may watch an interview being conducted or a surgical procedure being performed. Sometimes inferences about skill are made by observing outcomes, such as the absence of complications; but that analysis provides only a partial picture and the outcome may depend on other factors. (This multicausal model underlies the outcomes paradigm.) A more precise approach is first to ascertain what type of care produces the best (or at least acceptable levels of) results for a given problem (or group of patients). Then, one can apply the same deductive, analytic approach to examining those cases where the appropriate care was given to look for differences across providers. Where such differences are found, they can be said to reflect differences in skill.

HOW ARE OUTCOMES MEASURED?

Outcomes come in a variety of sizes and shapes. They can include familiar clinical measures, such as clinical signs and symptoms, or death. They can be expressed as complications, such as infections. But outcomes can also be couched in a larger context, which relies on patient-centered information often obtained by means of questionnaires. The selection of an outcome measure should be based on a clear sense of what one wants to measure and why. Outcome measures can be both generic and specific to a given problem. The generic measures are useful for looking at policy issues or reflecting the bottom-line effects of care on health status or even aspects of quality of life. They provide a sort of *lingua franca* that can be used to compare the treatments for various conditions in analyses such as cost-effectiveness.

Because much medical care can affect specific signs and symptoms but may not have a profound impact on the greater spheres of life, most clinicians are accustomed to looking at the more limited effects of care. These are more closely linked to specific interventions and, hence, are usually more satisfying to see. Condition-specific outcomes, as the name implies, will vary with the condition being treated, although some measures may prove useful for more than one condition.

Generic measures address larger constructs and, hence, their causal links to specific treatment events may be more difficult to trace. The generic measures can include both measures of function in various sectors (e.g., self-care, social activity, emotional state) as well as satisfaction with the care provided, the way it is provided, and perhaps even the setting in which it is provided. It is not always easy to separate opinions about the quality of care from feelings about the results of treatment. While someone may feel satisfied that a clinician did his or her best even if the results are disappointing, it is likely that patients will be more satisfied when the results are favorable.

As a basic rule of outcomes measurement, the more global the outcome measured, the more distant it is from the specific effects of the immediate treatment and the more sensitive it is to the effects of other intervening forces. Thus, measures of social role function are likely to be influenced by many factors other than the treatment of immediate interest. Isolating the role of treatment in the causal pathway will require controlling for many other variables, both around the time of treatment and subsequently. Alternatively, the analysis will rely on large numbers of observations, with the intent of detecting a relationship despite the noise the other factors may create.

Both generic and condition-specific outcomes measures (as well as the other components of the outcomes formula) often need to be aggregated to create some sort of summary measure. The aggregation process is complex. There is a strong temptation simply to add raw scores to generate a total score, but such a step is foolhardy. In the simplest case, it implies an equal weighting among the components, an assumption that is not automatically true. Even worse, the components may take on different weights because of the way the answers are constructed. For example, a response with five categories may receive a score of 1 to 5, whereas a dichotomous answer would be 0, 1. There is no *a priori* reason to suspect that a 5 on the first scale is any more important than a 1 on the second.

Aggregating multiple components of outcomes into a single bottom-line measure raises two important issues: (1) how to derive the weights to be applied to each component to reflect its relative importance and (2) what values to use in determining that importance. Many stakeholders may be involved, including patients and their families, the payers, the clinicians, and society.

Deciding how to weight the components of a summary scale properly can be a serious undertaking. Ordinarily, one needs some construct to use as the basis for norming the values placed on each component. Techniques that vary in sophistication and ease of implementation (usually inversely) can be applied to obtaining the value weights of different constituencies. In the outcomes trade, these values are usually referred to as *utility weights*. Sometimes they are directly related to overt concepts; sometimes they are inferred from observed behaviors.

The science of measurement has come a long way. Before an outcomes measure can be said to have attained its pedigree, it must pass a series of tests. Basically, the criteria for a useful measure are that it is reliable (i.e., it will yield the same results consistently), it is valid (i.e., it measures what it says it does), and it can detect meaningful increments of change.

Some measures have been extensively studied; others are more novel. Few, if any, can be used on all occasions. The astute outcomes researcher must weigh the measure's reputation against its actual content and the application intended. For example, some measures work well with some populations but not with others. They may cover only a limited portion of the full performance spectrum or be better at distinguishing among some aspects of function than others.

WHAT IS THE FIRST STEP?

A critical step in developing an outcomes study is the creation of a conceptual model. This need will be stressed frequently in this book because it is so central to successful outcomes work. In essence, the *conceptual model* indicates what is believed to cause the outcome. It should identify which variables, chosen to represent the various components of the basic outcomes equation described earlier, are pertinent to the study at hand. The variables themselves and their relationship both to the outcomes of interest and to each other should be specified.

A familiar saying in outcomes research is, "what cannot be measured does not exist." In one sense, the concept is attractive. It is necessary to be able to reduce complex attributes to measurable representations in order to study them and to compare their presence across programs. However, one must approach measurement with respect. Measurement involves distortion; it is by nature a process of abstraction, and something is inevitably lost in the process.

Likewise, the commitment to measurement should not be construed as endorsing the idea that everything that can be measured is useful. Perhaps one of the most memorable misuses of measurement was the theory behind the conduct of the Vietnam War. Body counts and arbitrary definitions of successful missions do not necessarily lead to a successful conclusion. Quantitative analysis works best when it serves conceptual thinking, not when it is a substitute for it. In his autobiography, Colin Powell describes an intelligence unit in Vietnam that received endless amounts of data on the enemy's shelling patterns. All this information was entered into a computer regression model that eventually produced the result that shelling was heavier on moonless nights, an observation that any combat veteran could have provided (Powell, 1995).

Outcomes research shares some of these problems. On the one hand, if its findings do not agree with clinical wisdom, they are distrusted. On the other hand, if they support such beliefs, they are extraneous. Life is generally too complicated to attempt outcomes analysis without some sort of framework. Some analysts may believe that the data will speak for themselves, but most appreciate the value of a frame of reference. Even more important, with so much information waiting to be collected, one needs some basis for even deciding where to look for the most powerful answers.

Using outcomes wisely requires having a good feel for what question is being asked and what factors are likely to influence the answer. Outcomes research is largely still a clinical undertaking, although it has become sophisticated. At its heart is a clinical model of causation.

Before an outcomes study can be planned, the investigator needs to develop a clear model of the factors that are believed to be most salient and their relationship to the outcomes of interest. Some factors will play a direct role; others may influence events more indirectly. Each needs to be captured and its role defined. This model forms the basis of the analysis plan.

A conceptual model is not necessarily the same as a theoretical model. No disciplinary theory needs to drive the model. Instead, it should explicate clearly what process the investigator believes is occurring, or at least what elements need to be controlled in the analysis. Such a model can be based on clinical experience as well as a review of prior work. Working the model through provides a way to think about what factors are most important. Figure 1–1 offers a simple illustration of a conceptual model for looking at the outcomes of congestive heart failure. The items in the boxes are operationalized aspects of the basic elements that are addressed in the outcomes formula described earlier. The arrows indicate an expected effect. In this model, the effects of treatment are expected to interact with the clinical factors to produce outcomes.

Once these elements have been identified, they can be operationalized. Each one can be captured in one or more measures. The delineation of the model and the specification of variables represent two of the major components of a research design. The third key ingredient is the analysis plan.[4] The conceptual model provides a general framework for the analysis, but the specifics will depend on several factors, primarily the nature of the variables. Most analyses, especially

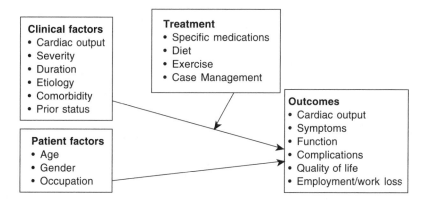

Figure 1–1 Conceptual Model of Treatment and Outcomes for Congestive Heart Failure

those that rely on an epidemiological approach, will have to be multivariate. One or another variation of regression models will likely be employed. Although multivariate modeling can take into account the effects of intervening variables, nonrandom assignment invariably raises questions about the comparability of treatment and control groups. Even groups that seem very comparable on the basis of variables examined may vary widely along some other parameter. Some researchers have proposed statistical models to deal with this so-called selection bias. Special models are developed to identify and deal with the correlated error associated with such a bias. These corrections usually use two levels of equations: one that describes care use and a second that estimates the outcomes for each type of care used. While many factors are common to both equations, one or more factors must be identified that are closely linked to utilization but not to the outcomes of that care, and vice versa.

Interpreting the results of regression equations can be complicated. Fundamentally, the major question is whether the independent variable of greatest interest (usually treatment) is significantly related to the dependent variable (i.e., the outcome) after the effects of other factors have been considered. This relationship can be examined in two ways: (1) the extent to which a change in the risk factor affects the dependent variable (e.g., the odds ratio) and (2) the capacity of the full equation to explain the variance in the model. It is quite feasible for a variable to be very significantly related to the dependent variable in an equation that explains very little of the overall variance. Conversely, explaining the variance does not examine the relationship between the independent variables and the dependent variable. In epidemiological terms, the size and strength of a coefficient from the regression equation reflect the power of the relationship, whereas the amount of variance explained describes the power of the overall model. It is possible to have a very significant relationship among variables and still not explain much of the total variance in the distribution of the dependent variable. Because outcomes may be influenced by many things, not all of them measurable, many outcome equations do not explain large amounts of the variance, although the adjusted relationship between variables of interest may be significant. Being able to establish a clear relationship between a treatment and its purported effects is important even when that relationship does not account for all, or even most, of the effect. A clear understanding of how a treatment influences outcomes for defined subgroups of patients lays the foundation for meaningful guidelines about what constitutes appropriate care.

HOW IS THIS BOOK ORGANIZED?

The rest of this book is organized to discuss the implications of the basic outcomes model. Each component is discussed at length to identify the issues that must be considered and to suggest some measures that may prove useful (along with caveats about using them). The book is divided into four parts, which correspond to the components of the outcomes equation.[5] The first part addresses outcomes measures, including generic measures, condition-specific measures, and satisfaction. The second part discusses treatment and proposes a taxonomy for this central component. The third part covers the major components of risk adjustment, including severity of illness, comorbidity, and demographic and psychosocial characteristics. The last part provides a somewhat technical discussion of measurement issues, and the final chapter offers some modestly practical[6] suggestions for those who are anxious to launch into outcomes studies. Although these observations are intended primarily for neophytes, it is hoped that they will provide some useful insights to experienced outcomes researchers as well.

REFERENCES

Donabedian, A. (1966). Evaluating the quality of medical care. *Milbank Memorial Fund Quarterly*, XLIV(3), 166–206.
Powell, C.L. & Persico, J.E. (1995). *My American journey*. (1st ed.). New York: Random House.

NOTES

1. Random assignment does not confer an absolute protection against bias. It simply reduces the likelihood that such bias has occurred. It is still important to examine the characteristics of the experimental and control groups to look for such bias and to consider the value of subgroup analysis where the effects of treatment may be greater with one portion of the sample than another.
2. Terminology varies a great deal with respect to the use of the term *risk factors*. Some people use it interchangeably with *disease severity*. Others use it more generically to refer to the whole set of

factors that can influence the outcomes of care (even including treatment). In this book, it is used consistently to refer to those factors other than treatment that can affect outcomes.

3. It would be possible to deal with clusters of diagnoses, but the numbers of combinations could quickly become unmanageable.

4. This book does not attempt to discuss the intricacies of the analytic methods for nonexperimental studies. Investigators should consult with a methodologist and/or statistician before any outcomes analysis is undertaken.

5. For the purposes of this discussion, baseline is not a separate entity because it is composed of the same measures used for outcomes.

6. Many would suggest that academics proposing practical insights constitutes an oxymoron!

Part I

Outcomes Measures

It seems self-evident that one cannot undertake outcomes research without developing useful measures of the outcomes. At first blush, the question of how to measure outcomes seems straightforward, but there is substantial dissention in the ranks. At least three distinct components of outcomes can be identified: (1) generic measures, (2) condition-specific measures, and (3) satisfaction. Each of these is discussed here in a separate chapter.

Historically, most clinical outcomes measures have been directed at specific diseases or problems, but, in the last two decades, attention increasingly has turned to using more generic measures that capture the ultimate effects of the clinical problems on the lives of patients (and their families). Each of these types of measure has its proponents and detractors. It makes good sense to expect that medical care should be assessed on the basis of its ultimate effects, but much of what is done on a daily basis likely does not achieve such profound consequences. While condition-specific measures are generally more satisfying to clinicians, who see a direct relationship between treatment and specific outcomes, others maintain that the true test of a treatment's effectiveness lies on a higher plane: its impact on relevant components of the patient's life.

This argument over whether generic measures are preferable to condition-specific ones seems unproductive. Each approach has strengths and limitations. Most outcomes studies will want to use elements of both. Indeed, there is even a movement afoot to merge the two approaches by seeking condition-specific measures of patient functioning.

One generic area of obvious concern is patient satisfaction. Patients are, and should be, the focus of medical efforts, but the extent to which patients' perceptions can be used as primary sources of judgments about the quality of care is debated. Increasingly, for both practical and theoretical reasons, patient satisfaction has become a central part of the spectrum of outcomes.

Patients can play several important roles in assessing quality. They are a source of important information. Some information can be obtained only from patients. For example, although observers may try to infer conclusions about a patient's pain and mood, only the patient can offer an accurate report. Patients are becoming more involved in decisions about their care. Consumer sovereignty is being recognized. Although patients may not have deep scientific knowledge about the efficacy of specific treatments, they are the best judges of what outcomes they want to maximize.

The same study may contain several outcomes. These outcomes can be analyzed separately, or some method of combining them can be employed. The way they are combined can, of course, influence the conclusions of the study. It is generally insufficient simply to add the various outcomes together. At a minimum, some sort of weighing process is needed to determine the relative importance of each outcome. Patient preferences should play a central role in this process, although some might argue that other interests (such as the payers' or society's) should also be represented. A number of methods are available to carry out the weighting procedure. They vary in both concept and complexity. In general, the most elegant are also the most abstract.

2

Generic Measures

Matthew Maciejewski

CHAPTER OUTLINE

- Why Use Generic Measures?
- How Do Researchers Plan Generic Measurement?
- How Do Domains of Health Relate to Outcomes Research?
- What Alternative Approaches to the Domains of Health Exist?
- What Are the Criteria for Good Generic Health Status Measures?
- From What Existing Measures Can Investigators Choose?

Two classes of measures can be used to assess outcomes: condition-specific measures and generic measures.[1]

Condition-specific measures (discussed in Chapter 3) focus on symptoms and signs that reflect the status of a given medical condition. They may also assess the direct sequela of a disease on a person's life. As a result, they are likely to be sensitive to subtle changes in health.

Generic measures, on the other hand, are comprehensive measures that assess overall effects on health status. These measures can be multidimensional or unidimensional and can be applied in different types of diseases, treatments, and patients. For example, the Sickness Impact Profile (SIP) has been used to evaluate physical and social health, and other domains, in rheumatoid arthritis, low back pain, and myocardial infarction patients (Deyo & Diehr, 1983; Deyo et al., 1982; Ott et al., 1983), and the 36-Item Short-Form Health Survey (SF-36) was used to compare the several chronic conditions studied in the Medical Outcomes Study (MOS); (Kravitz et al., 1992; Safran, Tarlov, & Rogers, 1994).

WHY USE GENERIC MEASURES?

In concert with the World Health Organization's definition of health (World Health Organization [WHO], 1948), generic health status measures are designed to capture physical, psychological, and social aspects of health. Clinicians who are interested in measuring a broad definition of health will find generic measures useful as bottom-line indicators of the effects of treatments on health status and quality of life. Generic measures can be used to measure health along the entire range of health from well-being to disability. These measures can augment laboratory tests and provider perceptions of patient health that focus on symptoms and signs of disease. Patient perceptions of social and psychological health and overall health status can be more accurate assessments than physician judgments in these domains.

Patient perceptions of health may be inconsistent with other measures of health (e.g., laboratory tests) because of response biases. Subjective responses to generic measures may reflect a patient's personality and disposition. Potential bias does not invalidate generic measures, it simply requires their careful use.

Health has been evaluated in terms of both quantity of health and quality of health. Many of the traditional outcome measures are based on counts of the frequency of occurrence of specific events that rely on definitional separations between function and dysfunction. These traditional measures tend to have face validity and to be measured across populations. Many of these generic quantity-of-health measures—mortality, morbidity, and average life expectancy—can be easily aggregated to provide summary figures that are easy to understand. Vital statistics rely on assessments of traditional health measures. Quality of health, on the other hand, reflects the importance or value attributed to overall health and functioning.

HOW DO RESEARCHERS PLAN GENERIC MEASUREMENT?

In order to measure health, a conceptual model must be developed to guide the choice of the appropriate aspects of health and range of dysfunction one wants to measure. A conceptual model is a framework for illustrating causal relationships. Physical functioning is the most common aspect of health that clinicians associate with the measurement of overall health. However, overall health in other domains is important in many clinical investigations.

Traditional Measures of Health

The simplest ways to assess outcomes across populations have been generic measures of mortality or health services utilization. Mortality and morbidity measures are generic measures that assess the quantity of health in a given population or across populations. Morbidity measures the presence of illness and the degree of dysfunction. Utilization of health services is sometimes used as a proxy for morbidity, although other factors beyond illness can influence use. If a narrow quantity of health measure is the only health outcome of interest, then a measure of mortality or morbidity may be the appropriate measure. These traditional measures are easy to interpret and compare across populations and time. However, quantity-of-health measures say little about the social or emotional functioning of a population. These measures tend to be crude endpoints.

Quality-of-Health Measures

Another set of generic measures is based on a richer but still restricted concept of health: health-related quality of life (HRQOL). HRQOL refers to the experience and importance of different domains of health that are affected by disease and treatment (Patrick & Erickson, 1993; Ware, 1995).[2] Five concepts define the scope of HRQOL: (1) impairments, (2) functional states, (3) health perceptions, (4) social opportunities, and (5) duration of life (Patrick & Deyo, 1989). These five concepts represent the different ways that dysfunction and treatment affect well-being and quality of life.

Domains or health constructs have been operationalized to translate these five concepts of quality of life into a measurable form. Domains of functioning vary in importance depending on the condition in question. Accurate and valid comparisons across patients or time require that the domains be the same in order to measure the same aspects of health.

Although there is no consensus about the inclusive set of domains, all investigators can agree that quality of life means different things to different people. This point has two implications. First, researchers may think about the domains of health in different ways. Different generic measures will capture different aspects of health based on different concepts of health. What is asked limits what is answered. Second, patients or survey respondents may value or weight various constructs differently. Researchers must decide whether to use measures that are weighted individually by each respondent or to assign weights to each question in a construct explicitly, according to some social weighting scheme. Thus, values play subtle but important roles at several levels in assessing health.

HOW DO DOMAINS OF HEALTH RELATE TO
OUTCOMES RESEARCH?

The five concepts of HRQOL provide a way of thinking about quality of life as it relates to well-being and health status. However, they are extremely general concepts that do not directly relate to observable aspects of patient health. The seven domains of health listed in Table 2–1 define these general concepts in terms of measurable, less abstract constructs. These domains represent a synthesis of alternative models of HRQOL. The seven domains are (1) physical functioning, (2) social functioning, (3) emotional functioning, (4) cognitive functioning, (5) pain, (6) vitality, and (7) overall well-being. For example, functional states can be assessed in physical, emotional, social, and cognitive domains. The five concepts of HRQOL overlap with domains of health, but there is not a one-to-one relationship. Health measured in a single domain may relate to several aspects of HRQOL.

Physical Functioning

Physical functioning refers to the range of an individual's mobility and independence in three types of physical ability: (1) fitness or physiologic health, (2) basic activity restrictions (activities of daily living [ADLs]), and (3) more advanced independent living restrictions (instrumental ADLs [IADLs]). Fitness is commonly assessed by moderate or vigorous physical exertions such as walking several miles or playing tennis. The ability to perform basic self-care ADLs, such as toileting, dressing, and feeding, are fundamental to an assessment of physical health status. ADLs are assumed to measure a hierarchy of physical functioning

Table 2–1 Seven Domains of Health

Domain	Examples of Possible Survey Items
Physical functioning	Range of motion of limbs, feeding and bathing, walking outdoors, shopping and cleaning
Social functioning	Visits with friends and family, restrictions on working, ability to babysit grandchildren
Emotional functioning	Feeling depressed or psychologically distressed, feeling happy
Cognitive functioning	Problems remembering important dates or events, awareness of current time and place
Pain/discomfort	Feeling bodily pain when getting out of bed, feeling aches when lifting even light objects, itching
Vitality	Lacking energy, feeling tired, needing to nap frequently
Overall well-being	Feeling satisfied with overall health, feeling content in general

based on Guttman scaling (Katz et al., 1963; Lazaridis et al., 1994). Greater self-sufficiency based on IADLs, such as shopping, writing, and cleaning, are also indicators of physical functioning. Together, these three sets of physical tasks represent the range of functionality (Kane & Kane, 1981). They form a crude hierarchy (Finch, Kane, & Philp, 1995). The specific choice of measure depends on the population addressed. Different sets tap different parts of the functional spectrum better.

Social Functioning

Social functioning captures the range of an individual's social interaction and interdependence in four ways: (1) social role limitations, (2) involvement in the community, (3) closeness of interpersonal relationships, and (4) coping. *Social role limitations* refer to an individual's ability to perform a social responsibility, such as mother or friend, to that individual's expectations. *Involvement in the community* refers to the network of family and friends that an individual comes into contact with on a regular basis. This involvement is a measure of the degree of integration with his or her environment, whereas social role limitations focus more on the person's performance in that network. The third aspect of social functioning—*closeness of relationships*—refers to the quality of the social network, as opposed to the quantity of contacts in the community. This concept reflects social support and the comfort derived from meaningful relationships. It is based on interdependence relative to other people, as is community involvement. *Coping* refers to the individual's ability to tolerate and maintain social relations while burdened with illness.

Emotional Functioning

Emotional functioning refers to an individual's range of affective well-being in terms of positive and negative emotions and the stability of emotions. For example, the SF-36 has a question about the amount of time the patient has been very nervous, happy, and downhearted (Ware & Sherbourne, 1992). The stability of emotions refers to the emotional fluctuations an individual undergoes over the course of an illness or treatment.

Cognitive Functioning

Cognitive functioning refers to an individual's range of intellectual ability in three ways: (1) memory, (2) reasoning abilities, and (3) orientation. The ability to remember significant dates and events in the past or future is a common measure of cognitive functioning, but thinking is a much more complex process. Several different generic measures test memory, including the Mental Status Questionnaire (Kahn et al., 1960). *Reasoning ability* refers to an individual's ability to do simple reasoning or computational tasks. Although these are best tested directly, it is possible to ask respondents to note problems they are experiencing in these areas. The SIP has a question asking the patient if he or she has trouble making plans, making decisions, or learning new things (Bergner, Bobbitt, & Carter, et al., 1981). *Orientation* captures an individual's awareness of current surroundings. Orientation (e.g., getting lost) is a common aspect of cognitive functioning queried in older adult patients.

Pain

The domain of pain assesses the degree of debilitating physical discomfort distinct from physical functioning. *Pain* commonly refers to bodily pain and itching experienced by an individual. Some people use other words to describe uncomfortable sensations, like *aches* and *cramps*. Headaches may not always be considered pain. Other types of discomfort may be even more annoying, such as itching. (People scratch to convert itching to pain.) Pain is assessed according to its intensity, duration, and frequency. Depending on the population and condition of interest, intensity and duration may be more important than frequency. For example, patients with chronic arthritis may constantly experience joint pain, with some episodes being more intense and longer than others.

Vitality

The degree of *vitality* that an individual feels is captured by two constructs: (1) energy and (2) sleep and rest. This domain includes positive and negative ranges of vitality. For example, two questions on the SF-36 ask if patients feel full of pep and if patients feel tired. Sleep is also included in this domain because an individual's vitality will be influenced by his or her amount of rest. Two questions on the SIP on sleep and rest ask patients if they sit during much of the day and if they sleep or nap during the day.

Overall Well-Being

Overall life satisfaction, or *overall well-being*, is a global evaluation of an individual's sense of contentment. This domain provides a comprehensive assessment of the patient's sense of his or her health status and happiness. In essence, overall well-being implicitly incorporates the physical, psychological, and social dimensions and their interactions. This domain is commonly assessed with broad questions asking patients about their overall health and well-being. The best known question used to assess overall health is, "In general, would you say your health is excellent, very good, good, fair, or poor?" Overall well-being is a useful domain to include in most studies because this deceptively simple question has been found to be a good predictor of mortality (Idler & Kasl, 1991; Mossey & Shapiro, 1982). Combined with the other domains of health, assessment of overall well-being can provide a complete conception of HRQOL.

WHAT ALTERNATIVE APPROACHES TO THE DOMAINS OF HEALTH EXIST?

These seven domains represent the multiple domains of health that investigators should consider in assessing quality of life. This model of the domains of health represents the simplest way to conceptualize health, but it is, by no means, the only way to define the domains of health.

The domains of health discussed here have been partitioned differently by various health services researchers. The different meanings attributed to HRQOL by different people have resulted in various conceptual models of health. Three alternative models of health domains are arranged in Table 2–2 according to the seven domains already presented. By grouping the other models according to the most general domains discussed here, the omissions and expansions in each model can be more easily identified. While each model covers most of the domains discussed, differences exist in how each domain is operationalized.

The Hall Model of HRQOL

Hall and colleagues (1989) have conceptualized the domains of health into seven distinct aspects that differ slightly from the model already discussed in this chapter. These seven domains are (1) functional health, (2) physiologic health, (3) social activity within the family, (4) social activity outside the family, (5) emotional health, (6) cognitive functioning, and (7) aggregate health. They hypothesized that these domains would be related to either physical health or psychosocial health. Their measures of functional health and physiologic health have physical functioning as a common denominator.

The domain of social functioning was similarly partitioned into two different dimensions. While both concepts capture social health in relationships, the first one is a measure of closeness with loved ones, and the second is a measure of

Table 2–2 Alternative Approaches to Domains of Health

Basic Domains	Hall, Epstein, & McNeil (1989)	Bergner (1989)	Ware (1995)
Physical functioning	Functional health; physiologic health	Physical functioning; symptoms	Physical functioning
Social functioning	Social activity with/ outside of family	Social functioning; role activities	Social functioning; role functioning
Emotional functioning	Emotional health	Emotional status; spiritual well-being	Psychological distress; well-being
Cognitive functioning	Cognitive functioning	Cognitive functioning	Cognitive functioning
Pain			Pain
Vitality		Energy and vitality; sleep and rest	Energy and fatigue; sleep
Overall well-being	Aggregate health	General health perceptions; general life satisfaction	General health perceptions; general life satisfaction

social networks. Cognitive and emotional health were modeled and assessed in a way similar to the basic model addressed previously.

The measure of aggregate health is similar to the concept of overall well-being. The conceptual model suggested by Hall and colleagues is similar to the model proposed earlier, but their model omits the important domains of pain and vitality.

The SIP Model of HRQOL

A more expansive framework for quality of life has been posited by Marilyn Bergner, one of the creators of the SIP. Her model of the quality of life domains includes the following: physical functioning, symptoms, social functioning, role activities, emotional status, cognitive functioning, energy and vitality, sleep and rest, general health perceptions, and overall life satisfaction (Bergner, 1989). Aspects of *physical functioning* assessed are self-care, mobility, and physical activity. Role activities are assessed according to work and household management. *Social functioning* includes aspects of personal interactions, intimacy, and community interactions. *Emotional status* is measured according to anxiety, stress, depression, locus of control, and spiritual well-being. Bergner's domains of role activities and social functioning contain aspects of health that were considered subsets of the aggregate health domain of social functioning. *Role activities* are social role activities, while *social functioning* refers to relationships at the personal and community levels. Bergner defines the aspects of *emotional status* in a similar manner to the basic conceptual domain, but she includes spiritual well-being as an aspect of emotional status that might otherwise be included in the domain of overall well-being.

The domain of health labeled *vitality* was partitioned by Bergner into *energy and vitality*, and *sleep and rest*. The domain of pain is not included in her conceptual model. The last domain of overall well-being has been partitioned into *general health perceptions* and *overall life satisfaction*. *General health perceptions* refer to the self-rated health question (from excellent to poor), while *general life satisfaction* refers to an overall evaluation of life beyond health. Both constructs have well-being as a common denominator that assesses health status and happiness. On the whole, Bergner's conceptual model of quality of life captures all but one domain of health (pain), but is more specific than the seven domains of health discussed earlier.

The Ware Model of HRQOL

The creators of the SF-36 have proposed the most comprehensive of all the alternative conceptual models. Twelve domains are included in their model: (1) physical functioning, (2) social functioning, (3) role functioning, (4) psychological distress, (5) general health perceptions, (6) bodily pain, (7) energy/fatigue, (8) psychological well-being, (9) sleep, (10) cognitive functioning, (11) quality of life, and (12) reported health transition (Stewart & Ware, 1992).

The physical functioning, cognitive functioning, and pain domains specified by Ware, Kosinski, and Keller (1996) are similar to the three domains of health discussed at the outset. The differences lie in the other categories of social functioning, emotional functioning, vitality, and overall well-being.

Emotional functioning is partitioned into two domains; psychological distress and psychological well-being. These two domains represent the negative and positive ranges of emotion, whereas the one domain of emotional functioning or emotional status accounts for the entire range in the other models.

Like Bergner, Ware and colleagues (1996) define two domains to capture vitality: energy and fatigue, and sleep. Vitality is assessed with questions about feeling worn out, tired, or full of pep. Sleep is assessed with questions about the amount of sleep. Overall well-being in the Ware model is composed of two distinct domains: general health perceptions and quality of life. This construct extends beyond general health perceptions and overall well-being to incorporate non–health-related factors.

The SF-36, one of the most popular generic instruments, was developed by Ware and colleagues and captures eight of these domains. These eight domains are parallel to the seven domains listed in the first column of Table 2–2, with the exception that physical functioning is separated into the domains of physical functioning and physical roles. The SF-36 is the 36-item short form of the 149-question Medical Outcomes Study Functioning and Well-Being Profile, which captures all 12 domains. An even briefer 12-item version has been developed that addresses all eight domains of the SF-36 (Ware et al., 1996). No existing measure captures all 12 domains in a short format.

Investigators must determine which domains are most salient to their population, condition, and question of interest. The conceptual model should guide the choice of domains. The multidimensional measures of quality of life can be used intact, or subscales can be employed as unidimensional measures.[3]

WHAT ARE THE CRITERIA FOR GOOD GENERIC HEALTH STATUS MEASURES?

The criteria for an ideal generic measure are listed in Table 2–3. They include conceptual issues, practical concerns, and psychometric properties. Most of the criteria apply to both unidimensional and multidimensional measures, but issues like weighting apply specifically to the latter. The relevance of each criterion to selecting the most appropriate generic measures follows.

Domains of Health

A conceptual model should dictate the quantitative and qualitative aspects of health to be measured. Most constructs of HRQOL involve multiple domains, but one domain or aspect may be more important. In this case, unidimensional measures may be more important. For example, ADLs may be the appropriate measure if physical functioning is paramount in a population of older adult patients. The domains salient to a particular condition or patient population should influence the choice of measure, not the other way around.

Multidimensional measures have the advantage of capturing health status across domains that may not have been expected by the investigator, but care must be taken to avoid the "kitchen sink" approach. Without a conceptual model, observing and reporting unexpected findings may exacerbate the perception of post hoc rationalization. Unidimensional measures are likely to be more sensitive to minor changes in that one domain, whereas an aggregated measure may dilute

Table 2–3 Criteria for Choosing a Generic Measure

Criterion	Impact on Measure
Domains of health	Choice of domains affects the treatment effects observed.
Range of health	Range of measure affects the coverage of the spectrum of performance and change in health status.
Clinical relevance	The interpretation of score will be difficult if numbers do not have a logical ordering and connection to reality.
Level of emphasis	The emphasis determines the relative weight of each domain in the measure.
Sensitivity	The inability of the measure to detect change in health status will miss important subtle changes.
Reliability	Unreliable measures yield inconsistent, uninterpretable results.
Validity	Valid measures provide information about the dysfunction of interest.
Practical considerations	The burden of administration influences the responses from patients and providers and amount of information obtained.

this effect. These trade-offs must be considered when determining which domains of health should be measured in a given investigation.

Range of Health

The range of health refers to the possible stages of dysfunction that patients may experience. Patient health lies on a continuum that spans from well-being to impairment to death (Institute of Medicine, 1992; Nagi, 1991; WHO, 1980). The following illustrates six points along the continuum of dysfunction:

Well-Being—Disease—Impairment—Functional Limitation—Disability—Death

Well-being, a concept first made prominent by the WHO, refers to a state of complete social, mental, and physical health. *Disease* refers to an interruption of bodily processes due to infection, trauma, or metabolic imbalance. *Impairment* is a greater degree of illness that results in "a loss or abnormality of an anatomical, physiological, mental, or emotional nature (Nagi, 1991, p. 315). *Functional limi-*

tations are characterized by manifestations at the level of the entire organism, not just dysfunction in an organ or one system. *Disability*, the stage prior to *death*, refers to an "inability or limitation in performing socially defined roles and tasks" (Nagi, 1991, p. 317).

Different measures capture different portions along the continuum. All measures are subject to floor and ceiling effects. A floor effect is the inability to measure health below a certain range. For example, the SF-36 is most sensitive to the health status effects of disease and impairment when healthy populations become ill. It does not do as well in distinguishing the very ill from the ill. Conversely, a ceiling effect is the inability to capture health above a certain range. ADLs may trace the loss of function, but saying that someone has no dependencies does not describe well just how functional he or she is. A conceptual model of the health status and disease will help to identify the suitable stages of dysfunction to be measured.

Clinical Relevance

Clinical relevance refers to the relationship between the health status domains in a generic measure and the expected path of patient dysfunction or recovery. Knowing the expected clinical course and potential adverse effects of both the disease and its treatments will help guide the choice of relevant measures. Mortality may not be clinically relevant for most clinical investigations in which death is not a likely occurrence (e.g., arthritis). Clinical relevance also refers to the usefulness of information derived from a measure. Results that can be translated into practice are more relevant than measures that are harder to interpret. Generic measures run the risk of being hard to put into a clinical context: what does a score of "x" on a scale of well-being mean?

Level of Emphasis or Dimensionality

Level of emphasis refers to the relative focus placed on different constructs or domains in an instrument. Essentially, this translates into the number of questions used to capture a certain construct. Most generic measures avoid levels of emphasis across several domains to address all domains equally. In some cases, the investigator may want to emphasize one or two domains over others because they are especially relevant to the problem being studied. For example, in a study of lower back pain, one may want to address physiologic functioning and pain in more detail. However, other domains, like social functioning, may also be relevant in a study of lower back pain. The relative focus that domains receive will be an important consideration in the choice of existing measures.

Sensitivity

The *sensitivity* of a measure refers to its ability to detect small changes in health across different patient populations. These changes can result from disease progression or the effects of treatment. In general, generic measures are less sensitive than disease-specific measures, or unidimensional measures. For example, the SF-36 asks general questions about pain but not about the intensity of pain. A more focused measure of pain would explore the location, intensity, nature, and duration of the pain. Issues affected by sensitivity are discussed more in Chapter 9.

Reliability

Reliability is a critical psychometric property that a good generic measure should demonstrate; it is virtually a precondition to its use. In psychometric terms, *reliability* has several meanings. For scales, *internal reliability* refers to the degree of concordance between any item and the overall scale score. Most reports of internal consistency for generic measures use Chronbach's alpha.[4] The statistic produces ranges from 0 to 1; the latter represents perfect internal consistency where all questions measure the same construct.[5]

A generic measure is said to be reliable if, on repeated administrations, consistent results are obtained. Reliability is commonly assessed by administering the same instrument to the same population at two points in time (*test–retest*) or by having two separate decision makers evaluate the same set of cases (*interrater*). Although this topic is discussed in more detail in Chapter 9, it is important to note here that reliability in one setting may not be equivalent to reliability in another. Especially in the context of interrater or test–retest reliability, the performance of one set of judges or respondents may not predict well how a different group will respond, particularly if the groups differ on relevant characteristics.

Validity

Validity indicates whether an instrument is measuring the constructs it was designed to measure. Testing validity is usually much more challenging than establishing reliability. The various ways to assess validity are addressed in Chapter 9.

Practical Considerations

In almost all cases, investigators are advised to use an extant generic health status measure (or portions of it) instead of trying to create one *de novo*. (The development work involved is extensive and would dwarf most applied studies.)

Several practical considerations must be addressed when choosing a generic health status measure. These practical issues should be considered once the conceptual model and psychometric issues are dealt with, not the other way around. These considerations include:

- the length of time required to administer the questionnaire
- the appropriate format for the survey (telephone, face-to-face, or self-administered)
- the use of proxy respondents
- the cost of administration (data collection and data entry)
- the complexity of the measurement and scoring methods
- the acceptability of the survey to patients/respondents and clinicians
- the expected format for presenting the results

Policy makers and clinicians generally find single, comprehensive values of health or quality of life more palatable than a set of scale values associated with different domains. (The simplicity of traditional generic measures, such as infant mortality or life expectancy, may partly explain their persistence in public policy analysis.) However, scores may not be meaningful per se. To get someone's attention, the score has to be understood in a context that is significant to the audience. Moreover, the same score may mean different things to different people. For those working actively with a scale, score values may become rectified as facts, but, for most people, they are not. Treating score values as indisputable, objective indicators of underlying health should be avoided.

Investigators must balance the burden of survey administration on interviewers and respondents with the breadth of health domains covered. Respondent attention will vary with the underlying nature of the respondents and the situation. Long questionnaires cannot be completed in a busy clinic while people are waiting to see the physician. Older adult or chronically ill populations may show problems of comprehension and/or fatigue. The time frame of a question can be important. There is often a trade-off between the time span needed to generate enough events and the accuracy of recall. Different types of information can be reliably remembered for various times. Questionnaires must be designed to minimize the difficulty in answering them. Pilot testing to ensure that the questions are interpreted as they were intended can prevent disastrous mistakes.

In many cases, the cost of survey administration will influence the choice of generic measure. As a general rule, complicated, high-quality data on patient quality of life will be expensive to collect. They usually require interviewers to administer the questions and interpret them or probe for further responses. New forms of interactive computerized interviews may reduce the need for interviewers, but several logistical issues must be resolved before this approach is widely available.

Last, the acceptability of the survey to patients and clinicians is important to ensure reasonable response rates. The Cooperative Information Project (COOP) Charts developed by Nelson and colleagues (1990) at Dartmouth are unique among multidimensional generic measures in accompanying survey questions by pictures associated with Likert-type responses. For example, a question about physical functioning has answers ranging from very little work to very heavy work with a picture of someone doing dishes as little work and someone running as very heavy work (Nelson et al., 1990). This intuitive format was highly acceptable to patients and clinicians. The results were also easily interpreted because the COOP Charts have only one question for each health construct. Investigators have to balance presentation of results and the psychometric properties of their measure. Surveys that use single measures may have deficiencies in validity and reliability. By contrast, the results from complex, multidimensional measures may provide results that require careful interpretation.

Each of these criteria should be considered for all measures, but all do not need to be satisfied before a generic measure can be considered useful. Often, it is a tradeoff between the ideal characteristics for a measure and the practicalities of application.

Preference Weighting

Having collected results of multidimensional scales, the investigator must struggle with how to combine them into a single, meaningful aggregated index. Both clinicians and policy makers are usually looking for some sort of bottom-line summary measure that captures the overall impact of the results. Some means of weighting the relative importance of the individual components is needed. Simply adding components without making any attempt to weight them does not escape the problem. Such addition uses an unstated equal weighting, which may be at least as biased as any attempt to apply more deliberate weights. *Preference*, or *utility weighting*, refers to placing value judgments on health states achieved or avoided by treatment (Sackett & Torrance, 1978). These weights reflect the relative importance of various states of health when compared with an anchor, such as perfect health or death. Preference-weighted summary measures are critical when performing cost-effectiveness and quality-adjusted life year calculations.

Both unidimensional and multidimensional health status measures must explicitly include preference weights in one way or another. However, weighting in multidimensional measures is given emphasis here because these measures commonly have a large number of questions across several domains that are more complicated to aggregate. Weighting is more straightforward in unidimensional measures, since several questions may be added together to obtain a single value for only one domain. For both types of generic measures, assessing preferences for different health states will improve the clinical relevance of index values.

Four steps are involved in conducting preference weighting: (1) choice of judges, (2) description of health states, (3) selection of measurement method, and (4) assignment of weights. There are four ways to measure preference weights, and each has its merits. Weights can be: arbitrarily assigned to questions, inferred from observations of social behavior, obtained from the literature on preference weighting, or derived through original data collection efforts (Patrick & Erickson, 1992). The fifth way to assign weights is really a variant of the first. Not overtly assigning weights to items (i.e., weighting each item equally) does not avoid the problem; it is as arbitrary as assigning specific weights.

Different people, or judges, may assign different values to each of the various states to be summed. The composition of the judging panel is as much a philosophical issue as a scientific issue. There are no fixed rules about whose opinions should be used. Potential raters include the patients themselves, care professionals, family members, regulators, policy makers, and the general public. In some cases, it is possible to allow each patient to provide his or her own value weights. When comparable measures are needed, a more consistent scheme of weighting is preferred. One can use a single source, or the weights can be calculated by combining the scores of different judges.

Arbitrary assignment of weights is the most common approach. A variant of the default approach in which all questions implicitly have equal weights makes an even graver error by using the direct weight of questions where the range of possible responses varies. Not only do the weights not reflect any theoretical value structure, they are based on a spurious factor. Collecting information on preference weights from population surveys is the most resource-intensive but may also be the most useful. Information derived from patients with experience with the illness under investigation may be different from that based on a sample of the general population, most of whom have had no direct exposure to the problem at hand.

A number of different methods have been developed for direct derivation of preference weights, including the standard gamble, time trade-off, psychophysical, and multidimensional methods (Froberg & Kane, 1989a, 1989b, 1989c, 1989d; Patrick & Erickson, 1992). Each of these methods requires careful consideration, and readers are advised to consult Froberg and Kane as an introduction. The accurate assessment of preference weights is important for cost-effectiveness studies and aggregation of generic measures into index scores. Investigators must determine the best way for their research problems; what they cannot afford is to ignore the issue.

FROM WHAT EXISTING MEASURES CAN INVESTIGATORS CHOOSE?

Health status measures have regularly addressed the four Ds—death, disease, disability, and discomfort—identified by Kerr White over three decades ago (White et al., 1961). Improved psychometric work has simply enabled more sophisticated measurement of these elements. Clinical investigators now have a variety of alternative generic measures that can be used as substitutes or complements to these traditional indicators of health.

Traditional Measures

The most commonly used measures—mortality, morbidity, and utilization—are frequently used because they are the most accessible from medical records, health departments, and hospital charts. Mortality is a useful endpoint when there is a reasonable expectation that the problem being studied has a chance of leading to premature death. Mortality is most meaningful if expressed as the proportion of deaths from a particular cause over a defined time interval. Mortality suffers from both floor and ceiling effect.[6] On the one hand, its absence says little about any other point on the continuum of dysfunction; on the other hand, it is hard to get worse.

Morbidity can be assessed in several ways. It may reflect the incidence or prevalence of a disease, or it may be assessed as days of work missed or bed disability days. Evaluations relying solely on morbidity measures may exclude important extremes in outcomes, such as excellent health or death. These types of floor and ceiling effects are a concern in any generic status measure. Morbidity usually focuses only on physical health, but it also can capture the consequences of mental health and work-related limitations. If a broader range of dysfunction and other domains of health are relevant, then morbidity is not as useful as other, more comprehensive measures (Kaplan et al., 1989).

Utilization of health services measures has been used as a proxy of health status. Utilization is difficult to interpret as a measure of health because of differences in access to services and other factors related to the population's utilization. Cultural and economic factors in the patient population of interest may distort the relationship between health and utilization data (Johnson et al., 1995; Meredith & Siu, 1995).

Unidimensional Health Status Measures

Generic health status measures that assess only one domain of health have been developed for use in quality-of-life assessments. *Unidimensional measures* can be

Table 2–4 Selected Unidimensional Measures

Measure	Domain of Health	Number of Questions	Focus of Questions
Katz Index of ADLs (Katz et al., 1963)	Physical functioning	6 Dichotomous questions to create a scale of dependency	Bathing, dressing, toileting, transfer, continence, feeding
Barthel Index of ADLs (Mahoney & Barthel, 1965)	Physical functioning	10 Questions on performance based on 100-point scale	Feeding, grooming, toileting, walking, climbing stairs, continence
Comprehensive Older Person's Evaluation (Pearlman, 1987)	Physical functioning	100 Questions	Using telephone, handling money/personal items, keeping house, making meals
Zung Self-Rating Depression Scale (Zung, 1965)	Emotional function	20 Questions ranked 1–4 each that sum to 80	Feeling blue, lonely
Zung Self-Rating Anxiety Scale (Zung, 1971)	Emotional function	20 Questions ranked 1–4 that sum to 80	Feeling more nervous than usual; sleep easily
Mental Status Questionnaire (Kahn et al. 1960)	Cognitive function	10 Questions that sum to 10	Orientation based on current date, location, birthday
RAND Social Health Battery (Donald & Ware, 1984)	Social function	11 Questions	Social resources and contacts in family and community
MOS Social Support Survey (Sherbourne & Stewart, 1991)	Social function	20 Questions	Emotional support, informational support, tangible support, positive social interaction, affection

either a single indicator based on one question or a single index based on a summation of several questions tapping the same domain. For example, the Mental Health Inventory is a 5-question survey of mental health that is part of the SF-36, but can be used independently as a unidimensional measure. See Table 2–4 for selected unidimensional measures.

ADLs and IADLs are two measures that capture a single domain of health—physical functioning. The PULSES Profile (Moskowitz & McCann, 1957) and the Functional Activities Questionnaire (Pfeffer et al., 1982) are two additional measures of physical function for use in elderly populations. The Change in Function Index is a general physical functioning measure that can be used in adult populations (MacKenzie et al., 1986). Discussions of ADL and IADL measures of physical functioning, as well as selected measures of emotional, cognitive, and social functioning follow.

The health domain of emotional functioning also can be measured with an array of unidimensional measures. The Zung Self-Rating Anxiety and Self-Rating Depression Scales have all been developed to assess psychological and emotional functioning (Kane & Kane, 1981). Cognitive functioning can be assessed using the Mental Status Questionnaire (Kahn et al., 1960). Unidimensional measures of pain, vitality, and overall well-being are not discussed here; clinicians interested in measures of these domains should refer to the review by McDowell and Newell (1996).

One of the earliest measures of physical functioning—ADLs—was developed by Katz and colleagues in 1963 to assess basic concepts of self-care. A fairly standard set of activities is now used to assess patients' degree of independence or capacity for self-care, including dressing, bathing, using the toilet, transferring in and out of a bed/chair, and feeding. Two ADL scales—the Katz Index and the Barthel Index—are widely considered the best-known and validated measures of physical functioning. A third, the Functional Independence Measure (FIM) is widely used in the rehabilitation arena (Granger et al., 1993; Keith et al., 1987).

In its original form, trained raters administer the six questions in the Katz Index using detailed statements about each activity. Based on the description of bathing (e.g., sponge bath, tub bath, or shower), a patient is rated either independent (without assistance or assistance with only one part of the body) or dependent (assistance with more than one part of the body). An overall score ranges from fully dependent to fully independent in all activities, based on a ranking of activities in order of dependence. The ranking of activities from smallest loss of independence to greatest loss is bathing, dressing, toileting, transferring, continence, and feeding (Katz et al., 1963). Patients are considered less than fully independent if they cannot do any one of the activities, less independent still if they cannot bathe but do one additional activity, and further dependent as they do fewer activities. This schema has been found to be a reliable and valid measure of physical functioning. It is now commonly used as a self-administered questionnaire.

The Barthel Index uses a 100-point scale (Mahoney & Barthel, 1965) to create a weighted measure of the self-care activities of feeding, grooming, bathing, toileting, walking, climbing stairs, and continence (control of bladder and bowels). The Barthel Index is designed to be administered by medical staff. This hierarchical index is novel because each activity has a value associated with dependence or independence that sums to 100 for independence in all activities. In addition, continence is broken out into two dimensions, and walking and climbing stairs are added as basic elements of self-care. This measure also has been found to be a valid and reliable measure of physical functioning, primarily in older or more chronically ill patients. Like the Katz Index, the Barthel Index is a good predictor of mortality and hospitalization.

Investigators can assess a higher level of physical functioning by measures of the IADLs. These activities commonly include cooking, cleaning, doing laundry, shopping, using transportation, keeping track of money, taking medications, and using the telephone. Each of these activities requires a greater level of skill and mobility than the basic self-care concepts captured in ADLs.

Although numerous other measures have been developed, only one IADL measure—the Comprehensive Older Person's Evaluation (COPE) scale—is discussed here. The items in the COPE scale include using the telephone, handling money, securing personal items, tidying up, and preparing meals (Pearlman, 1987). The measure is designed to be administered by medical staff, who ask 100 questions of the patient that can be summed to 100 in an overall IADL score. When a measure of ADLs and a measure of IADLs is used, a broad range of physical functioning can be assessed. They can be combined into a single continuous scale (Finch et al., 1995).

Important issues in using ADL measures are the consistency in measures across settings (e.g., hospital, home) and formats (e.g., self rating, direct observation). The information obtained from the same survey questions has been shown to vary by setting and format (Dorevitch et al., 1992; Myers, 1992; Myers et al., 1993). Self-rated functioning was found to be closer to observations made directly by clinicians than was functioning rated by formal and informal caregivers (Dorevitch et al., 1992). Clinicians can underestimate the difficulty of several IADL tasks when compared with the self-rated evaluations by patients (Myers et al., 1993). Clinicians have to consider these and other sources of response bias when administering any measures of quality of life and functioning.

Emotional functioning can also be assessed independent of other measures, as in the case of ADLs for physical functioning. Unidimensional measures of emotional functioning tend to focus on a range of either positive or negative emotions (e.g., depression) to the exclusion of the other end of the continuum. Some measures, however, such as the Zung Self-Rating Depression Scale, include questions about depressive symptoms as well as optimism or fulfillment (Zung, 1965). The Zung Self-Rating Depression Scale is a self-administered survey of 20 questions that group into four general categories: (1) well-being, (2) depression, (3) optimism, and (4) symptoms (Blumenthal, 1975). Each question has a response ranging from "a little of the time" (score of 1) to "most of the time" (score of 4). The score is computed by adding the answers from each of the 20 questions.

A score below 50 indicates normal emotional functioning. A score between 51 and 56 indicates borderline depression, while any score above 56 indicates significant clinical depression.

The Zung Self-Rating Anxiety Scale is a similar unidimensional measure that assesses the presence and severity of affective and somatic symptoms related to clinical anxiety (Zung, 1971). The Zung Anxiety Scale also is a 20-question survey with each question ranked from 1 to 4. In this scale, a score of 44 or less indicates normal emotional functioning, while a score of 45 to 55 is a mark of significant anxiety. Severe anxiety is indicated by scores of 56 or above.

The Mental Status Questionnaire (MSQ) is a unidimensional measure of cognitive functioning based on orientation. The MSQ has been administered in the National Health and Nutrition Examination Survey to older adult respondents. This interviewer- or self-administered survey contains 10 questions about the date, location, the person's birthday, and the current and previous U.S. president (Kahn et al., 1960; Patrick & Erickson, 1992). The answers to these 10 questions are scored by giving 1 point for each correct answer. The overall, unweighted score is then divided into three categories: no cognitive dysfunction (0–2 errors), moderate dysfunction (3–8) errors, and severe dysfunction (9–10) errors. The MSQ has been found to be highly reliable in terms of both internal consistency and test–retest reliability. However, the MSQ does not break down cognitive functioning into other spheres, such as remote memory or reasoning abilities. The Philadelphia Geriatric Center (PGC) Extended MSQ, developed by Lawton, is a fuller version of the MSQ that includes several questions about more distant events to test remote memory (Kane & Kane, 1981; Lawton, 1968). Questions about remote memory include the names of the patient's mother and father. This version of the MSQ rounds out aspects of cognitive functioning but does not capture all aspects of cognitive functioning that may be pertinent to different clinical populations. There is some evidence that the levels of performance need to be adjusted for education and race. Since it was designed to be used primarily with older adults, it may not be as useful in younger groups.

A widely used, more comprehensive cognitive measure is the Multidimensional Mental Status Examination (MMSE) developed by Folstein and colleagues (1985). As its name implies, it taps a variety of dimensions of cognitive functioning, including spatial recognition. It can be administered by a modestly trained individual and has been used effectively in a variety of cultures but, again, some adjustments for education should be made in interpreting the results.

Any unidimensional measure of social functioning, such as the RAND Social Health Battery (Donald & Ware, 1984), should cover aspects of social role limitations, involvement in the community, closeness of interpersonal relationships, and coping. The RAND Social Health Battery is an 11-item, self-administered scale that was used in conjunction with the Health Insurance Experiment. The battery queries social functioning related to family and community life

(Donald & Ware, 1984). For example, one question asks the patient how many close friends he or she has. The RAND Battery demonstrated reasonable reliability in both internal consistency (0.68) and test–retest (0.68) terms but lower validity. While the RAND measure does not have strong psychometric properties, it is a short, easily administered social functioning measure.

An alternative unidimensional scale is the Social Support Survey constructed for use in the MOS (Sherbourne & Stewart, 1991). This 20-item self-administered survey covers five areas of social functioning: (1) emotional support, (2) informational support, (3) tangible support, (4) positive social interaction, and (5) affection. This measure has demonstrated high reliability (0.97) and validity. This unidimensional survey is also short and easy to administer and builds on earlier work by RAND and others.

Most unidimensional measures of social and cognitive functioning are based on work in psychiatry instead of the older, sociology-based measures presented above. Clinicians interested in these domains of health should refer to empirical literature that explores these aspects of health more fully.

Multidimensional Health Status Measures

A wide range of multidimensional measures that captures two or more domains of health is available to investigators. The following major measures are reviewed here:

- the 36-Item Short-Form Health Survey (SF-36)
- the Sickness Impact Profile
- the Nottingham Health Profile
- the Duke–University of North Carolina Health Profile
- the Quality of Well-Being Scale
- the Dartmouth COOP Charts

Table 2–5 lists these multidimensional measures and the domains they cover.

The SF-36

The SF-36 (Ware & Sherbourne, 1992) was developed to capture multiple domains of health across the entire continuum of health status (McHorney, Ware, & Raczek, 1993). It is, however, most useful in generally healthy populations.

As noted previously in this chapter, eight domains of health are measured by the SF-36. The physical functioning scale is a 10-item set of questions that capture the presence and extent of physical limitations. Questions query patients about lifting

Table 2–5 Domains Covered by Selected Multidimensional Measures

	Physical Functioning	Emotional Functioning	Cognitive Functioning	Social Functioning	Pain	Vitality	Overall Well-Being
SF-36	✓	✓		✓	✓	✓	✓
SIP	✓	✓	✓	✓	✓		✓
NHP	✓	✓		✓	✓	✓	
DUKE	✓	✓	✓	✓	✓	✓	
QWB	✓			✓		✓	
COOP	✓	✓		✓			✓

Key:
SF-36 = 36-Item Short-Form Health Survey (Ware & Sherbourne, 1992).
SIP = Sickness Impact Profile (Bergner, et al., 1981).
NHP = Nottingham Health Profile (Hunt, McKenna, & McEwen, 1980).
DUKE = Duke–University of North Carolina Health Profile (Parkerson, Broadhead, & Tse, 1990; Parkerson et al., 1989).
QWB = Quality of Well-Being Scale (Kaplan et al., 1989).
COOP = Dartmouth COOP Charts (Nelson & Berwick, 1989).

and carrying groceries, bending and kneeling, walking moderate distances, and other ADL-type functions. Role functioning is measured using a four-item scale for limitations due to physical problems and a three-item scale for limitations due to emotional problems. Bodily pain is measured by a two-item scale that asks about the frequency of bodily pain/discomfort and the extent of interference with normal activities due to pain.

Mental health is captured using the five-item Mental Health Inventory developed for the MOS (Ware & Sherbourne, 1992). Four mental health conditions are tapped: (1) anxiety, (2) depression, (3) loss of behavioral/emotional control, and (4) psychological well-being. Vitality, in terms of energy and fatigue, is measured using a four-item scale. Social functioning is measured using two questions that ask about physical and emotional health-related effects on social activities. Last, general health perceptions are assessed using a five-item scale that queries patients about self-perceived health.

These eight scales can be scored independently into easily interpreted patient evaluations. The SF-36 scales are not meant to be aggregated into a global or overall assessment of patient health, although they commonly are. Aggregation across scales blurs the distinctions within each domain of health that the measure was designed to tap. The purported strength of the SF-36 is the number of domains that it measures and the relatively broad range of health that it covers. However, the measure works best to distinguish states of illness from wellness. It is not as effective in distinguishing changes in dysfunction among those already disabled.

Reliability, content validity, and construct validity have been evaluated in numerous studies, and the SF-36 has been found to be highly reliable and valid for diverse patient groups and individuals (McHorney et al., 1993, 1994). Validity was assessed according to both psychometric and clinical criteria. To keep the health survey brief enough to be useful in clinical settings, certain domains of health were omitted. The SF-36 does not capture cognitive functioning. If this domain of health is relevant to the patient population and/or medical condition of interest, the SF-36 can be used in conjunction with other measures or can be replaced with one of several measures that do capture this domain.

Sickness Impact Profile

The SIP was developed at the University of Washington to provide a measure of health status sensitive enough to detect changes in health status over time or between groups (Bergner et al., 1981). This enables comparisons across types and severities of medical conditions and across demographic and cultural subgroups. The SIP consists of 6 domains, which are further divided into 12 subdomains of health. The six domains are physical functioning, emotional functioning, social functioning, cognitive functioning, pain, and overall well-being. These domains are divided into sleep and rest, eating, work, home management, recreation and pastimes, ambulation, mobility, body care and movement, social interaction, alertness behavior, emotional behavior, and communication.

The SIP contains 136 statements that are used to produce a percentage score for each of the 12 subdomains. The statements are divided unevenly among the 12 subdomains but can be summed to obtain an overall assessment of health status. In addition, a physical index score can be obtained by combining body care and movement, ambulation, and mobility scale scores. A psychosocial index score can be obtained by combining the emotional behavior, social interaction, and communication scale scores. Statements about sleep and rest include, "I sleep or nap during the day," whereas eating is assessing with statements such as, "I am eating special or different foods." Work is assessed with statements such as, "I am not working at all." Home management includes statements such as, "I am not doing heavy work around the house." Social interaction is assessed by statements such as, "I isolate myself as much as I can from the rest of the family." Communication is assessed with statements such as, "I do not speak clearly when I am under stress."

Reliability and validity of the SIP have been demonstrated in a number of field trials and in subsequent comparative analyses of generic measures. In a series of three field trials early in its development, the SIP obtained high reliability with Cronbach's alphas of 0.94 and above (Bergner, 1993). Validity in these three field trials was also found to capture accurately patient dysfunction and to correlate higher with clinical ratings of dysfunction than clinical ratings of sickness. In a study of patients with head injury, the SIP was found to correlate highly with neurologic and neuropsychologic severity indices (Temkin et al., 1989).

One of the strengths of the SIP is that it covers a large number of domains and subdomains of health-related quality of life. In addition, the SIP is sensitive to a wide variety of conditions and patient populations. The two greatest limitations to the SIP are its length and the omission of the vitality domain. At 136 statements, the SIP is one of the longer generic surveys. The breadth of domains covered is commendable, but the length of the instrument makes it impractical for use in most clinical investigations or practice settings. One way to overcome the problem of length is to use subsets of the SIP. The SIP omits the health domain of vitality from the survey, a critical domain for many patient populations and conditions. Overall, the SIP is a comprehensive alternative to the SF-36 if more detailed scale scores for a large number of subdomains are desired. Not only can the SIP provide scale scores for each of the 12 subdomains, but index scores for physical and psychosocial functioning can be obtained along with a composite or overall health status score. The various levels of aggregation are unique to the SIP. Care must be taken to combine scales according to the methods detailed by Bergner and colleagues (Bergner, 1993).

In response to the perceived need for a shorter version of the SIP, de Bruin and colleagues developed the SIP68, a 68-item version of the SIP. The SIP68 covers six *subdomains* to provide reliable and valid results in a less burdensome format (de Bruin et al., 1994a, 1994b). The six subdomains of the SIP68 are (1) somatic autonomy, (2) mobility control, (3) psychological autonomy and communication, (4) social behavior, (5) emotional stability, and (6) mobility range (Post et al., 1996). *Somatic autonomy* refers to basic ADLs. *Mobility control* refers to hand and arm control and basic control over one's body (de Bruin et al., 1994b). *Psychological autonomy and communication* measures cognitive functioning and one's ability to communicate. *Social behavior* refers to social functioning, and *emotional stability* refers to emotional functioning. Last, *mobility range* refers to IADL-type activities of shopping and personal business affairs. These six subdomains predicted scores from the original, 136-item SIP nearly perfectly ($R^2 = 0.96$). Although further testing and validation of the SIP68 remain to be done, early results indicate that it is a valid and reliable generic measure without the burden of the longer version.

Nottingham Health Profile

The Nottingham Health Profile (NHP), developed in England, covers all domains of health except cognitive functioning and overall well-being (Hunt et al., 1980). The NHP is a two-part instrument with a total of 45 questions. The first part consists of a 38-item survey that asks patients about physical functioning, vitality, pain, and emotional and social functioning. Vitality is subdivided into questions about sleep and energy (McEwen, 1993). The second part of the NHP includes seven questions about the problems caused by the patient's present state of health in seven areas: job or work, home management, social life, home life, sex life, interests/hobbies, and holidays.

The NHP was tested for face, content, and criterion validity (see Chapter 9 on Measurement) in its assessment of physical, social, and emotional domains of health. Validation studies have been done on older adult patients, general practice clinic patients, patients with peripheral vascular disease, and patients with non-acute conditions. In addition, reliability has been demonstrated in studies of patients with osteoarthritis and patients with peripheral vascular disease (McEwen, 1993). The NHP has been primarily used in clinical studies and population surveys in Europe.

The strengths of the NHP are: ease of administration, ease of interpretation, usefulness as a measure of general health status in a variety of conditions and populations, and high reliability and validity. These strengths are similar to those in the SF-36 and SIP, but the NHP provides an alternative approach to health because it focuses on the departure from health. Because the NHP was developed in England, it has a slightly different cultural foundation. Nonetheless, it has been successfully incorporated into studies in the United States.

The limitations of the NHP include the possibility of false positives due to the severity of dysfunction used in survey questions and its focus on the negative aspects of health as opposed to concepts of well-being and positive health. The first limitation is a potential problem in many patient populations where sensitivity to minor health changes is important. Despite these limitations, the NHP has been shown to be valid and reliable across several domains of health. The range of domains covered and its distinct cultural heritage provide sufficient reasons to consider its use in quality-of-life investigations.

Duke Health Profile

A longer, 63-item version of the Duke–University of North Carolina Health Profile (DUHP) measures symptom status, physical functioning, social functioning, and emotional functioning. On further application in clinical trials, the longer survey was found to have several conceptual problems that led to difficulties in scoring and interpretation of scales (Parkerson et al., 1989, 1990). Self-esteem was the only indicator of emotional health, and social role performance was the only measure of social functioning. These unidimensional constructs do not assess the presence *and* extent of dysfunction in these two domains of health.

To correct for these conceptual problems and to provide a shorter, more practical survey instrument, Parkerson and colleagues created the 17-item Duke Health Profile (DUKE) (Parkerson, Connis et al., 1993). This generic measure was constructed to maintain the convergent and discriminant validity of the larger DUHP as well as high internal consistency and test–retest reliability. Clinical validity was also assessed to determine how well the DUKE survey could distinguish between patients with different types of physical and mental health problems.

The physical health of patients was assessed by questions using ADL-type measures of sleeping, walking up a flight of stairs, and running. Mental health was assessed by questions such as self-perceived depression and nervousness. A patient's social health was captured by questions about family relationships, involvement in family and social groups, and other factors. These questions demonstrated reasonably good reliability, with Cronbach's alpha values between 0.55 to 0.78, and reasonable test–retest correlations (Parkerson et al., 1990). Psychometric and clinical validity were not as strongly validated. Much more extensive validation for this measure is necessary, a task that Parkerson and colleagues have begun to pursue (Broadhead, Parkerson, & Tse 1991; Parkerson et al., 1993).

One of the great strengths of the Duke health survey is its brevity. However, this brevity also compromises the psychometric properties of reliability and validity. This measure, and its longer predecessor, are comprehensive measures that may prove useful in many investigations after more testing in different patient populations and diagnostic groups. More work is necessary to ensure that the benefits of using this measure are not eclipsed by the costs of unreliable and uninterpretable results.

Quality of Well-Being Scale

The Quality of Well-Being Scale (QWB) is a 38-item generic measure that can be used to assess three domains of functioning: physical functioning, social functioning, and vitality (Kaplan et al., 1989). The QWB was the primary quality-of-life instrument used to rank health states in Oregon's health reform effort. Four scales capture the entire continuum of health from death to optimal functioning, which is uncommon among most of the widely used measures. This is achieved by combining mortality and morbidity into a single, comprehensive score (Kaplan, Anderson & Ganiats, 1993). Overall health from death to optimal functioning is evaluated by aggregating the three scale scores in a linear function to obtain values ranging from death at 0.0 to optimal health at 1.0. The QWB can be used to obtain point-in-time assessments of health status as well as projections of health using "well-years." An overall wellness score can be obtained from the QWB by aggregating subscales and converting them to well-years. *Well-years* integrate mortality and morbidity into health status in terms of well-years of life (Kaplan et al., 1993).

Utility weights are used to combine responses from the various questions into a single score. The QWB does not weight all questions equally but assigns negative weights according to the degree of dysfunction associated with a given question. The scale starts at 1.0 for optimal health, and responses to the survey shift the score away from optimal health as dysfunction is indicated. For example, three questions in the Social Activity Scale asking patients about major role limitations, minor role limitations, and other role limitations are weighted –0.061. The utility weights were validated on a general population sample in San Diego, California. The generalizability of the weights has been demonstrated in a study of rheumatoid arthritics (Balaban et al., 1986).

The QWB has been used in a wide range of clinical studies, but validation studies comparing this measure to others have yet to be done. This generic instrument has been used in studies of rheumatoid arthritis, coronary artery bypass grafts, antihypertensive medications, acquired immunodeficiency syndrome (AIDS), and cystic fibrosis (Kaplan et al., 1989; Orenstein et al., 1990; Bombardier et al., 1986; Weinstein & Stason, 1985). Validity and reliability for this measure have not been thoroughly explored, a point that Kaplan and colleagues acknowledge (Kaplan et al., 1989). This sort of validation is necessary before the QWB can be used with confidence with conditions and populations different from those already examined.

Dartmouth COOP Charts

The COOP Charts developed as part of the Cooperative Information Project at Dartmouth were devised as generic measures that suited the clinical setting by satisfying five practical criteria:

1. Produce reliable and valid data on a range of domains.
2. Fit into routine office practice.
3. Apply to a range of illnesses.
4. Yield easily interpretable results.
5. Provide the clinician with useful information of patient functioning (Nelson & Berwick, 1989).

The COOP Charts employ a unique format of survey presentation. Each question about a given domain of health, for example, physical functioning, is accompanied by pictures associated with responses. These charts are used to assess the domains of physical, emotional, and social functioning, as well as overall well-being. The nine charts focus on physical, emotional, role, and social functioning; overall health; and change in health, pain, overall quality of life, and social support (Nelson et al., 1990). Each of the charts provides five possible answers and is not meant to be aggregated.

Convergent and discriminant validity has been assessed by comparing responses from COOP Charts and the health survey used in the RAND Health Insurance Experiment. The COOP Charts were validated with patients in four outpatient settings: (1) patients in primary care clinics, (2) elderly patients in

Veterans Affairs (VA) clinics, (3) hypertensive and diabetic patients in university hospital clinics, and (4) patients with chronic diseases in several sites in the MOS. High convergent validity was demonstrated using the multitrait-multimethod technique (Nelson et al., 1990). Reliability was assessed by surveying patients two times with a 1-hour interval and with a 2-week interval. High reliability was demonstrated in the 1-hour interval, but much lower reliability was found in the 2-week interval. Nelson and colleagues argue that health status in patients visiting a physician's office should change markedly over a 2-week period, so low 2-week reliability should not be a concern. The COOP Charts are a novel approach to evaluating health with generic measures.

Future research should be conducted using COOP Charts in populations with a range of illnesses, both acute and chronic, not captured in earlier work. The patient and clinician acceptance of the nine COOP Charts was quite high, and their practicality did not entirely sacrifice validity and reliability. This measure, however, omits several potentially important domains of health (e.g., cognitive functioning, pain, and vitality).

CONCLUSION

The evaluation of health status and health-related quality of life often deserves greater consideration than may seem necessary at first. Careful attention to conceptualization of health domains and an exact definition of quality can facilitate the valid and reliable assessment of patient health. Four main points can serve as guidelines:

- Generic measures are the best way to capture multidimensional aspects of health. These types of measures are designed to assess patient health across several domains (physical/social/emotional/cognitive functioning, pain, vitality, and overall well-being). Measures may obtain a single index number from values in separate domains, such as the SIP, or may obtain individual values for each domain. In either case, generic measures are the ones to use if overall patient health is the desired outcome.
- It is best to determine which of the seven domains are salient to your problem, and then choose the generic measure that captures those domains. Each measure will have one or more questions that focus on a specific aspect of functioning, and different measures incorporate different combinations of domains. No single measure will work best in all possible patient populations and medical conditions. Choosing the measure appropriate for one's study is a critical first step in effective outcomes research.
- Generic measures should be collected at baseline (as well as follow-up) to indicate where a patient's course began. The measurement of health status to

indicate improving or worsening health is only meaningful if a before–after comparison can be made. Otherwise, only point-in-time evaluations can be made.

- The more easily understood the measure, the more useful it is. Generic measures generally have life anchors to relate a numeric value to a state or condition of health. In other words, results based on scale scores need to be placed in the context of daily life to be easily interpreted. The values obtained from a generic measure must have a clinical context to be useful sources of information.

REFERENCES

Balaban, D.J., Sagi, P.C., Goldfarb, N.I., & Nettler, S. (1986). Weights for scoring the quality of well-being instrument among rheumatoid arthritics. *Medical Care, 24*, 973–980.

Bergner, M. (1989). Quality of life, health status, and clinical research. *Medical Care, 27*(3), S148–S156.

Bergner, M. (1993). Development, testing, and use of the Sickness Impact Profile. In Walker, S.R. & Rosser, R.M. (Eds.), *Quality of life assessment: Key issues in the 1990s* (pp. 95–111). Boston: Kluwer Publishing.

Bergner, M., Bobbitt, R.A., Carter, W.B., & Gibson, B.S. (1981). The sickness impact profile: Development and final revision of a health status measure. *Medical Care, 8*, 787–805.

Blumenthal, M.D. (1975). Measuring depressive symptomatology in a general population. *Archives of General Psychiatry, 32*(8), 971–978.

Bombardier, C., Ware, J., Russell, I.J., Larson, M., Chalmers, A., & Reed, J.L. (1986). Auranofin therapy and quality of life for patients with rheumatoid arthritis: Results of a multicenter trial. *American Journal of Medicine, 81*, 565–578.

de Bruin, A.F., Buys, M., DeWitte, L.P., & Diederiks, J.P. (1994a). The sickness impact profile: SIP68, A short generic version. First evaluation of the reliability and reproducibility. *Journal of Clinical Epidemiology, 47*(8), 863–871.

de Bruin, A.F., Diederiks, J.P., DeWitte, L.P., Stevens, F.C., & Philipsen, M. (1994b). The development of a short generic version of the sickness impact profile. *Journal of Clinical Epidemiology, 47*(4), 407–418.

Deyo, R.A., & Diehr, P. (1983). Measuring physical and psychosocial function in patients with low back pain. *Spine, 8*, 635.

Deyo, R.A., Inui, T.S., Leininger, J., & Overman, S. (1982). Physical and psychosocial function in rheumatoid arthritis: Clinical use of a self-administered health status instrument. *Annals of Internal Medicine, 142*(5), 879–882.

Donald, C.A., & Ware, J.E.J. (1984). The measurement of social support. *Research in Community and Mental Health, 4*, 325–370.

Dorevitch, M., Cossar, R., Bailey, F., Bisset, T., Lewis, S.J., & Wise, L.A. (1992). The accuracy of self and informant ratings of physical capacity in the elderly. *Journal of Clinical Epidemiology, 45*, 791–798.

Finch, M., Kane, R.L., Philp, I. (1995). Developing a new metric for ADLs. *Journal of the American Geriatrics Society, 43*(8), 877–884.

Folstein, M., Anthony, J.C., Pahad, I., Duffy, B., & Gruenberg, E.M. (1985). The meaning of cognitive impairment in the elderly. *Journal of the American Geriatrics Society, 33*, 228–233.

Froberg, D.G., & Kane, R.L. (1989a). Methodology for measuring health-state preferences—I: Measurement strategies. *Journal of Clinical Epidemiology, 42*(4), 345–354.

Froberg, D.G., & Kane, R.L. (1989b). Methodology for measuring health-state preferences—II: Scaling methods. *Journal of Clinical Epidemiology, 42*(5), 459–471.

Froberg, D.G., & Kane, R.L. (1989c). Methodology for measuring health-state preferences—III: Population and context effects. *Journal of Clinical Epidemiology, 42*(6), 585–592.

Froberg, D.G., & Kane, R.L. (1989d). Methodology for measuring health-state preferences—IV: Progress and a research agenda. *Journal of Clinical Epidemiology, 42*(7), 675–685.

Granger, C.V., Hamilton, B.B., Linacre, J.M., Heinemann, A.W., & Wright, B.D. (1993). Performance profiles of the functional independence measure. *American Journal of Physical Medicine and Rehabilitation, 72*, 84–89.

Hall, J.A., Epstein, A.M., & McNeil, B.J. (1989). Multidimensionality of health status in an elderly population. *Medical Care, 27*(3), S168–S177.

Hunt, S.M., McKenna, S.P., & McEwen, J.A. (1980). A quantitative approach to perceived health status: A validation study. *Journal of Epidemiology and Community Health, 34*, 281–285.

Idler, E.L., & Kasl, S. (1991). Health perceptions and survival: Do global evaluations of health status really predict mortality? *Journal of Gerontology, 46*(2), S55–S65.

Institute of Medicine. (1992). *Guidelines for clinical practice: From development to use.* Washington, DC: National Academy Press.

Johnson, P.A., Goldman, L., Orav, E.J., Garcia, T., Pearson, S.D., & Lee, T.M. (1995). Comparison of the medical outcomes study short-form 36-item health survey in black patients and white patients with acute chest pain. *Medical Care, 33*(2), 145–160.

Kahn, R.L., Goldfarb, A.I., Pollack, M., & Peck, A. (1960). Brief objective measures for the determination of mental status in the aged. *American Journal of Psychiatry, 117*, 326–328.

Kane, R.A., & Kane, R.L. (1981). *Assessing the elderly: A practical guide to measurement.* Lexington, MA: DC Heath.

Kaplan, R.M., Anderson, J.P., & Ganiats, T.G. (1993). The quality of well-being scale: Rationale for a single quality of life index. In Walker, S.R. & Rosser, R.M. (Eds.), *Quality of life assessment: Key issues in the 1990s,* (pp. 65–95), Boston: Kluwer Publishing.

Kaplan, R.M., Anderson, J.P., Wu, A.W., Mathews, W.C., Kozin, F., & Orenstein, D. (1989). The quality of well-being scale: Applications in AIDS, cystic fibrosis, and arthritis. *Medical Care, 27*(3), S27–S43.

Katz, S., Ford, A.B., Moskowitz, R.W., Jackson, B.A., & Jaffee, M.W. (1963). Studies of illness in the aged: The index of ADL: A standardized measure of biological and psychosocial function. *JAMA, 185*, 914–919.

Keith, R., Granger, C., Hamilton, B., & Sherwin, F. (1987). The functional independence measure: a new tool for rehabilitation. In Eisenberg, M.G. & Grzesiak, R.C. (Eds.), *Advances in Clinical Rehabilitation: Vol. 1* (pp. 6–18). New York: Springer-Verlag.

Kravitz, R.L., Greenfield, S., Rogers, W., Manning, W.G. Jr., Zubkoff, M., Nelson, E.C., Tarlov, A.R., & Ware, J.E., Jr. (1992). Differences in the mix of patients among medical specialties and systems of care: Results from the medical outcomes study. *JAMA, 267*(12), 1,617–1,623.

Lawton, M.P. (1968). The PGC mental status questionnaire [mimeograph]. Philadelphia: Philadelphia Geriatric Center.

Lazaridis, E.N., Rudberg, M.A., Furner, S.E., & Cassel, C.K. (1994). Do activities of daily living have a hierarchical structure? An analysis using the longitudinal study of aging. *Journal of Gerontology: Medical Sciences, 49*(2), M47–M51.

MacKenzie, C.R., Charlson, M.E., DiGioia, D., & Kelley, K. (1986). A patient-specific measure of change in maximal function. *Archives of Internal Medicine, 146*(7), 1,325–1,329.

Mahoney, F.I., & Barthel, D.W. (1965). Functional evaluation: The Barthel index. *Maryland State Medical Journal, 14*, 61–65.

McDowell, I., & Newell, C. (1996). *Measuring health: A guide to rating scales and questionnaires.* New York: Oxford University Press.

McEwen, J. (1993). The Nottingham health profile. In Walker & Rossi (Eds.), *Quality of life assessment: Key issues in the 1990s* (pp. 111–130). Boston: Kluwer Publishing.

McHorney, C.A., Ware, J.E., Lee, J.F.R., & Sherbourne, C.D. (1994). The MOS 36-item short-form health survey (SF-36): III. Tests of data quality, scaling assumptions, and reliability across diverse patient groups. *Medical Care, 32*(1), 40–66.

McHorney, C.A., Ware, J.E. Jr., & Raczek, A.E.. (1993). The MOS 36-item short-form health survey (SF-36): II. Psychometric and clinical tests of validity in measuring physical and mental health constructs. *Medical Care, 31*(3), 247–263.

Meredith, L.S., & Siu, A.L. (1995). Variation and quality of self-report health data: Asian and Pacific Islanders compared with other ethnic groups. *Medical Care, 33*(11), 1,120–1,131.

Moskowitz, E., & McCann, C.B. (1957). Classification of disability in the chronically ill and aging. *Journal of Chronic Disease, 5*, 342.

Mossey, J.M., & Shapiro, E. (1982). Self-rated health: A prediction of mortality among the elderly. *American Journal of Public Health, 72*, 800–808.

Myers, A.M. (1992). The clinical Swiss Army knife: Empirical evidence on the validity of IADL functional status measures. *Medical Care, 30*(5), MS96–MS111.

Myers, A.M., Holliday, P.J., Harvey, K.A., & Hutchinson, K.S. (1993). Functional performance measures: Are they superior to self-assessments? *Journal of Gerontology: Medical Sciences, 48*(5), M196–M206.

Nagi, S.Z. (1991). Some conceptual issues in disability and rehabilitation: Appendix A. In Pope, A.M. & Tarlov, A.R. (Eds.), *Disability in America: Toward a national agenda for prevention* (pp. 309–327). Washington, DC: National Academy Press.

Nelson, E.C., & Berwick, D.M. (1989). The measurement of health status in clinical practice. *Medical Care, 27*(3), S77–S90.

Nelson, E.C., Landgraf, J.M., Hays, R.D., Wasson, J.M., & Kirk, J.W. (1990). The functional status of patients: How can it be measured in physicians' offices? *Medical Care, 28*(12), 1,111–1,126.

Nunally, J.C., & Bernstein, I.M. (1994). *Psychometric Theory* (3rd ed.). New York: McGraw–Hill.

Orenstein, D.M., Pattishall, E.N., Nixon, P.A., Ross, E.A., & Kaplan, R.M. (1990). Quality of well-being before and after antibiotic treatment of pulmonary exacerbation in cystic fibrosis. *Chest, 98*, 1,081–1,084.

Ott, C.R., Sivarajan, E.S., Newton, K.M. (1983). A controlled randomized study of early cardiac rehabilitation: The sickness impact profile as an assessment tool. *Heart and Lung, 12*(2), 162–170.

Parkerson, G.R., Broadhead, W.E., & Tse, C.J.K. (1990). The Duke health profile: A 17-item measure of health and dysfunction. *Medical Care, 28*, 1,056.

Parkerson, G.R.J., Connis, R.T., Broadhead, W.E., Patrick, D.L., Taylor, T.R., & Tse, C.K. (1993). Disease specific versus generic measurement of health-related quality of life in insulin dependent diabetic patients. *Medical Care, 31*(7), 629–639.

Parkerson, G.R.J, Broadhead, W.E., & Tse, C.K.J. (1991). Development of the 17-item Duke health profile. *Family Practice, 8,* 396.

Parkerson, G.R.J, Michener, J.L., Wu, L.R., Finch, J.N., Muhlbaier, L.M., Magruder-Habib, K., Kertesz, J.W., Chapp-Channing, N., Morrow, D.S., Chen, A.L., et al. (1989). Association among family support, family stress, and personal functional health status. *Journal of Clinical Epidemiology, 42,* 217.

Patrick, D.L., & Deyo, R.A. (1989). Generic and disease-specific measures in assessing health status and quality of life. *Medical Care, 27*(3), S217–S232.

Patrick, D.L., & Erickson, P. (1992). *Health status and health policy.* New York: Oxford University Press.

Patrick, D.L., & Erickson, P. (1993). *Health status and health policy: Quality of life in health care evaluation and resource allocation.* New York: Oxford University Press.

Pearlman, R.A. (1987). Development of a functional assessment questionnaire for geriatric patients: The comprehensive older person's evaluation (COPE). *Journal of Chronic Disease, 40,* S85.

Pfeffer, R.I., Kurosaki, T.T., Harrah, C.H., Chance, J.M., & Filos, S. (1982). Measurement of functional activities in older adults in the community. *Journal of Gerontology, 37,* 323.

Post, M.W.M., de Bruin, A.F., DeWitte, L.P., & Schrijvers, A. (1996). The SIP68: A measure of health-related functional status in rehabilitation medicine. *Archives of Physical Medicine and Rehabilitation, 77*(5), 440–445.

Sackett, D.L., & Torrance, G.W. (1978). The utility of different health states as perceived by the general public. *Journal of Chronic Diseases, 31,* 697–704.

Safran, D.G., Tarlov, A.R., & Rogers, W.M. (1994). Primary care performance in fee-for-service and prepaid health care systems: Results from the MOS. *JAMA, 271*(20), 1,579–1,586.

Sherbourne, C.D, & Stewart, A.L. (1991). The MOS social support survey. *Social Science and Medicine, 32,* 705–714.

Stewart, A.L., & Ware, J.E.J. (Eds.). (1992). *Measuring functioning and well-being.* Durham: Duke University Press.

Temkin, N.R, Dikmen, S., Machamer, J., & McLean, A. (1989). General versus disease-specific measures: Further work on the Sickness Impact Profile for head injury. *Medical Care, 27*(3), S44–S53.

Ware, J.E. Jr. (1995). The status of health assessment, 1994. *Annual Review of Public Health, 16,* 327–354.

Ware, J.E. Jr., Kosinski, M., & Keller, S.D. (1996). A 12-item short-form health survey: Construction of scales and preliminary tests of reliability and validity. *Medical Care, 34*(3), 220–233.

Ware, J.E. Jr., & Sherbourne, C.D. (1992). The MOS 36-item short-form health survey (SF-36). I. Conceptual framework and item selection. *Medical Care, 30*(6), 473–483.

Weinstein, M.C., & Stason, W.B. (1985). Cost-effectiveness of interventions to prevent or treat coronary heart disease. *American Review of Public Health, 6,* 41–63.

White, K.L., Williams, T.I., & Greenberg, B.G. (1961). The ecology of medical care. *New England Journal of Medicine, 265,* 885–892.

World Health Organization. (1948). *Constitution of the World Health Organization: Basic documents.* Geneva, Switzerland: Author.

World Health Organization. (1980). *International classification of impairments, disabilities, and handicaps.* Geneva, Switzerland: Author.

Zung, W.W.K. (1965). A self-rating depression scale. *Archives of General Psychiatry, 12,* 63–70.

Zung, W.W.K. (1971). A rating instrument for anxiety disorders. *Psychosomatics, 12,* 371–379.

NOTES

1. Generic health measures may also be used as independent measures on occasion. The presence of a generic state in one domain may affect the likelihood of finding a generic outcome in another domain. Usually the generic measures used this way are collected at baseline, but they may also be contemporaneous with the outcome of interest. For example, being depressed may influence how a person reports his or her overall health status.
2. The term *HRQOL* is used in an effort to restrict discussions of quality of life to the aspects where health care can be reasonably expected to play some role. For example, having friends or earning a large income is not expected to be a realistic goal for good care.
3. Multidimensional measures assess two or more domains while unidimensional measures focus solely on one domain.
4. Chronbach's alpha is an estimate of the expected correlation of one test with an alternative form containing the same number of items (Nunally and Bernstein, 1994).
5. One would not actually want a state of perfect internal consistency because then each variable would add nothing new to the overall score.
6. A floor effect is a value that observations cannot fall below. A ceiling effect is a value that observations cannot exceed (Nunally and Bernstein, 1994).

3

Condition-Specific Measures

Adam Atherly

CHAPTER OUTLINE

- What Are the Differences between Condition-Specific and Generic Health Status Measures?
- What Drives the Choice of a Condition-Specific Measure?

The previous chapter discussed the use of generic health status measures in the measurement of outcomes. Health services researchers successfully have used generic health status measures to measure outcomes in a wide variety of settings. However, generic health status measures are only one alternative available to the outcomes researcher; condition-specific health status measures offer both advantages and limitations compared to their generic cousins. In using either, collecting baseline data is important in interpreting the results.

WHAT ARE THE DIFFERENCES BETWEEN CONDITION-SPECIFIC AND GENERIC HEALTH STATUS MEASURES?

Condition-specific outcomes measures are designed to measure changes in the most important domains of a specific condition. Condition-specific measures are available for many different diseases and afflictions. There are essentially two types of condition-specific measures: (1) clinical (which use primarily signs, symptoms, and tests) and (2) experiential (which capture the impact of the disease or problem on the patient, often in ways akin to those used in generic measures).

One definition is: "Condition-specific health status measures are measures designed to assess specific diagnostic groups or patient populations, often with the goal of measuring responsiveness or 'clinically important' changes" (Patrick and Deyo, 1989, p. s217).

Condition-specific measures are designed to be extremely sensitive to the detection of small treatment effects. Generic measures may fail to detect small changes for a number of reasons. First, condition-specific measures are designed to tap the domains of greatest interest for a particular condition. Generic health status measures, in contrast, cast a broad net across different facets of health. For example, the 36-Item Short-Form Health Survey (SF-36) measures across a broad spectrum; it attempts to tap eight conceptually separate aspects of functioning and mental well-being (Ware & Sherbourne, 1992). The numbers of variables in each domain vary from 2 to 10, which illustrates both a strength (breadth) and a weakness (i.e., minimal coverage of any single domain) of a broad health status measure. The SF-36 may be able to tap several different dimensions of an intervention that is expected to affect health in a variety of ways. For example, certain drugs may improve physical functioning while causing fatigue. A generic health status measure could evaluate both of these effects. However, this breadth and flexibility is also a weakness of the generic health status measures.

Why Not Use Generic Health Status Measures?

According to Patrick and Deyo (1989, p. s217), "Generic health status measures purport to be broadly applicable across types and severities of disease, across different medical treatments or health interventions and across demographic and cultural subgroups." The generic health status measures may not isolate the variable(s) of greatest interest. For example, the SF-36 may not be a good choice to evaluate the effect of an intervention designed to help control pain. Because only two of the 36 questions deal with pain, much of the information provided by the SF-36 may be irrelevant (this is called *low content validity*). By not isolating the dimensions of greatest interest, a true treatment effect can be masked. In contrast, a condition-specific measure can be specifically designed to assess pain and can focus directly on the precise area of interest.

This focus is important not just to enable measures to be concise but to ensure that the health status measure is sensitive to clinically important differences or changes in health status. Determining whether or not a given treatment had an effect requires that the estimated effect is both statistically significant and clinically significant. Statistical significance, which refers to the likelihood that a result occurred by chance, is determined by such factors as the sample size and variance. The clinical significance of the treatment effect must be determined by the investigator.

A generic health status measure may miss clinically significant treatment effects for several reasons. First, there may be a "floor" or "ceiling" effect. A scale is considered to have a *ceiling effect* when individuals who are rated as perfectly healthy by the scale can be found to have health problems on other scales (Bombardier et al., 1995); the converse is a *floor effect*. For example, the SF-36 is designed to be used to assess the health status of reasonably healthy populations. If the SF-36 was used to assess the effect of an intervention on a population of frail older adults, the scale might miss a true treatment effect because the entire sample was bunched at the lower end of the scale both before and after the intervention. The condition-specific measure can be aimed at the proper part of the distribution (i.e., avoid ceiling and floor effects).

The second reason a generic health status measure may miss a clinically significant treatment effect is that it lacks sensitivity (Kessler & Mroczek, 1995). For some illnesses, a successful treatment may not result in an increase in the scores of an overall health status measure. For example, generic health status measures were insensitive to positive health changes resulting from successful treatment of benign prostatic hyperplasia—changes successfully measured by condition-specific measures (Barry et al., 1995).

More importantly, generic health status measures may simply fail to tap the necessary dimensions of health. For example, a successful treatment for hypertension would not necessarily affect the scores of a self-administered generic health status measure such as the SF-36. Yet, the successful treatment of the hypertension has a profound influence on the long-term health of the individual.

Condition-Specific Health Status Measures

A condition-specific measure can successfully tap the domains of greatest interest, but this advantage comes at a price. Condition-specific measures have several drawbacks. In order to measure a given condition more precisely, condition-specific measures cast a far narrower net than do generic measures. As a result, some unanticipated (or anticipated in a separate domain) effects from an intervention could be missed (Bombardier et al., 1995).

There is a second drawback associated with condition-specific health status measures: it is generally more difficult to compare the results of a study to those of other studies when condition-specific measures are used. In many settings, the investigator is not merely interested in finding a treatment effect, but also in estimating the importance of the treatment effect. If the investigator finds a 3-point increase in the Arthritis Impact Measurement Scales (AIMS) (Kazis, Anderson, & Meenan, 1989), what does this mean clinically? One possibility is to compare the findings to previous studies. However, for most conditions, a plethora of scales is available. If the investigator is concerned not merely with finding the presence of a treatment effect, but also in comparing the treatment with other similar studies, a condition-specific measure may complicate that comparison (although there are techniques available to aid in that task) (Guyatt, Feeny, & Patrick, 1993). Generic health status measures provide a common metric for comparisons across treatments, conditions, or populations.

Condition-specific outcome measures have another strength: they are often intuitively appealing, especially to clinicians. If one wishes to investigate the impact of a treatment on arthritis, a common-sense approach is to use a scale that specifically taps the dimensions of health affected by arthritis. The ultimate goal of outcomes research is to provide insights that lead to greater efficiency and higher quality of care. To have an impact on the delivery of care, the researcher must be able to persuade the medical care community that the findings are truly reflective of reality rather than simply a theoretical abstraction.

An excellent example of the strengths and limitations of the two types of measures was provided in a study of patients who underwent cataract surgery (Damiano et al., 1995). This study used both a generic health status measure (the Sickness Impact Profile [SIP]) (Bergner et al., 1976) and a vision-specific measure (the VF-14) (Steinberg, et al., 1994) to evaluate the impact of the surgery. A postoperative improvement in visual acuity was found to be unrelated to the SIP score; conversely, the VF-14 was found to be highly sensitive to changes in visual acuity. The authors conclude that the SIP is simply not sensitive enough to measure changes such as those caused by cataract surgery. However, the SIP did provide interesting insights. Several behaviors measured by the SIP that were not expected to be related to vision, such as "I act irritable and impatient," were found to be highly correlated with presurgery, better-eye visual acuity. This suggests that vision may affect health in ways not detected by a vision-specific measure.

Almost all measures of complications are condition specific. By definition, a complication of treatment is an untoward outcome associated with the treatment of a condition. Therefore, a complication is necessarily condition specific. (This is discussed in more detail in Chapter 7.)

Other Alternatives

Although a discussion of the use of condition-specific health status measures versus the use of generic health status measures is useful, the best alternative often is to try to combine the two approaches. The generality of the generic measures is both their strength and weakness; the generic measures exhibit breadth but not depth. The generic measures are able to find treatment effects across many domains but may fail to focus intently enough on the domains of most interest. Conversely, the condition-specific measures exhibit great depth but little breadth.

One obvious alternative is simply to use both a condition-specific measure *and* a generic measure (as in the Damiano et al. [1995] study mentioned previously).

If resources permit, this strategy is probably the best alternative. This was the course followed by Bombardier et al. (1995) in a study of pain and physical function after knee surgery. Among patients who reported knee pain, a generic measure (the SF-36) was unable to distinguish patients in need of knee surgery; the knee–pain-specific measure (the Western Ontario and McMaster Universities Osteoarthritis Index [WOMAC]) was able to do so. After surgery, patients often recovered enough that the WOMAC was unable to distinguish among patients, although some were extremely disabled, whereas the SF-36 was able to do so.

If it is necessary to use a single instrument, two approaches are available. First, a generic instrument can be modified for a specific condition. For example, an (unsuccessful) attempt was made to modify the SIP to make it more sensitive to head injury (Temkin et al., 1989). Items deemed nonapplicable were removed, and items believed particularly applicable to head injury were added. The scale was then reweighted. In this case, the modified SIP was no more effective than the unmodified SIP, so it was discarded. One drawback of this approach is that the strength of generic measures is the ability to compare to other studies that have used the same measure. Once a scale has been modified and reweighted, it is no more comparable to the original than a completely unrelated condition-specific measure.

Second, a generic instrument can have a condition-specific supplement attached to it. The goal of this approach is to have the condition-specific supplement not overlap measurement of the domains covered by the generic measurement but, instead, to expand more deeply into domains of particular interest (Patrick & Deyo, 1989). This approach retains the comparability of the generic measurement (since the measure is retained unchanged) and taps the domains of greatest interest in the supplement.

A final alternative is to use a battery of condition-specific measures. Since one of the major shortcomings of condition-specific measures is their narrowness and specificity (Kessler & Mroczek, 1995), the use of several different condition-specific tests may be an option. For example, Kjerulff and Langenberg (1995), in a study examining fatigue among patients having hysterectomy, used four different fatigue measures—Symptom Fatigue Scale, Profile of Mood States (McNair, Lorr, & Droppleman, 1971), and two scales from the Medical Outcomes Study Short-Form General Health Survey (Stewart, Hays, & Ware, 1988). Although each of the four scales ostensibly measured the latent construct "fatigue," each provided separate insights into how fatigue was affected by hysterectomy. *Fatigue* was broken down into three separate components: frequency of fatigue, the extent to which fatigue is problematic for the respondent, and the extent to which fatigue causes limitation of activity. The correlation of the components was high, but each predicted different events. For example, the extent to which fatigue is problematic was the best predictor of the number of physician contacts. Each scale contained unique information, and the authors of this study suggested that measurement of all three components is necessary for a complete analysis of fatigue.

Table 3–1 summarizes the options for using condition-specific measures, either alone or in combination.

WHAT DRIVES THE CHOICE OF A CONDITION-SPECIFIC MEASURE?

The Conceptual Model

Simply choosing the "best" measure available for a given condition from a statistical perspective is inadequate. The choice of a particular condition-specific measure should be guided more strongly by the investigator's conceptualization of what the condition-specific measure *ought* to measure rather than by narrow statistical guidelines.

The first step in picking a measure is to understand the natural history of the disease and to construct a theory regarding precisely how the intervention will affect the condition. With that model in place, available condition-specific measures can be evaluated to find one that taps the exact domain where the intervention is expected to have an impact.

In many cases, a disease can affect the life of an individual in many distinct ways. More importantly, a *single* disease can affect *multiple* domains of a single

Table 3–1 Ways To Use Condition-Specific Measures

Option	Discussion
Use a condition-specific and a generic measure.	Administering two different measures is potentially costly; otherwise, this is best option.
Modify generic measure.	A modified measure is not comparable with an unmodified measure; lose main advantage of generic measure.
Attach condition-specific supplement to generic measure.	Solid option. Retains comparability of generic measure. Necessary to find or develop supplement.
Use battery of condition-specific measures.	Pick condition-specific measures that tap all domains of interest. May be easier, cheaper, and more thorough to use generic and condition-specific measures. Battery does not retain the easy comparability of generic measures.

ill person's life. The selection of appropriate domains to study is the key to the selection of an appropriate condition-specific health status measure. As Kessler and Mroczek remind investigators, the selection of the domains is a difficult task: "The first issue that has to be confronted in selecting outcome measures concerns the appropriate domains. This is an easy issue to address in the abstract, because the researcher usually wants to measure all domains that might be importantly affected by the medical intervention under investigation. It is much more difficult to determine what these domains are in practice, however, because the intervention effects can be complex" (1995, p. AS109).

One way to conceptualize this issue is to consider the types of information that can be drawn from a study participant regarding the nature of his or her ailment. A health status measure can be thought of as evaluating symptoms, signs, tests, or functions. (See Table 3–2.)

A *symptom* would be something reported by the patient but not confirmed by other scientific means. Symptoms are typically the easiest and lowest cost type of event to measure; investigators simply need to ask the patient (Sherbourne & Meredith, 1992). There are some domains, like pain, that are very difficult (although possible) to measure in other ways.

Symptoms are inherently subjective. There is a prejudice against using subjective patient opinions; patient opinions are not considered to be as scientific as opinions rendered by trained medical professionals. The major difficulty with symptoms is establishing validity. For example, many different health questionnaires ask patients to rate their own level of pain. What precisely does this measure? Is it compared to the worst pain imaginable? The worst pain the individual has ever felt? The worst pain felt recently? The level of pain the individual typically feels? The level of pain the individual fears he or she might feel? Self-reported health measures are strongly influenced by such factors as ethnicity (Meredith & Siu, 1995) and social class (Koos, 1954). One example of

---

Table 3–2 Measurement by Condition-Specific Measures

	Definition	Example
Symptoms	Events reported but not confirmed by other means	Pain
Signs	Results reported by medical professional	Heart murmur
Test	Objective, reproducible finding by medical professional	Blood pressure
Function test	Measurement of item related to condition but not condition itself	Test of patient's ability to walk up stairs

this is the classic study of the relationship between culture and pain, which showed that individual responses to pain depend on social, family, and culturally patterned responses (Zborowski, 1952).

However, it is not clear that symptoms reported by patients are, in fact, less reliable than other types of measures. Symptoms have inherent face validity. Moreover, patient feelings can provide unique insights. For example, studies of self-reported health have found that it is one of the best available predictors of mortality (Idler & Kasl, 1991). The problem may be less one of lower actual validity than one of lower perceived validity.

A *sign* is a result reported by a medical professional after a direct examination of the patient. Signs are opinions expressed by medical professionals. For example, a physician listening to a patient's heart may report hearing a heart murmur. Signs are typically considered more valid than symptoms, although this may be a result of professional prejudice rather than empirical truth. The validity and reliability of a professional opinion are dependent on such factors as the training of the professional, the focus and quality of the instrument, and the level of ambiguity of the topic (Feinstein, 1977).

A *test* is an objective finding by a medical professional, such as a laboratory test. A test is typically considered to be superior to symptoms and signs because of better validity. When a population is tested for a disease, for example, the exact same procedure and exact same criteria can be used for every single member of the population. Every member of the population can give a blood sample of the same size. Every blood sample can be treated in the same way. The exact same antibody threshold can be used every time. With tests, extremely high validity can be established.

Tests are considered more valid than signs or symptoms. Again, however, this may be due to professional prejudice rather than true relationships. With many tests, interpretation of the results is necessary. For example, with an echocardiogram, after the test is complete, a medical professional needs to interpret the ultrasonic record. The ultrasonic record is shown as shadows on a monitor. The rater must make a judgment about the presence of potential anomalies. The quality, reliability, and validity of the test therefore depends entirely on the quality, reliability, and validity of the interpretation.

Another example of this is found in radiology. The rate of correct interpretations of mammograms of patients with cancer was between 74% and 96% (Elmore et al., 1994). The correct interpretation rate for patients without cancer ranged from 89% to 35%. Tests can be just as fallible as symptoms or signs.

Although one may feel confident in using a direct physiological measure as an outcome, even the simplest measure can produce unforeseen problems. For example, blood pressure seems like a straightforward parameter, but even as simple a measure as this can be presented in many ways. The way the variable is defined can affect the result and even dramatically alter the interpretation. An analysis by Berlowitz and his colleagues showed that depending on how blood pressure was used (e.g., last diastolic blood pressure [DBP] determination ≥ 90, mean DBP over 1 year), the relative performance of clinical sites changed (Berlowitz et al., in press).

Finally, a *function test* does not attempt to measure aspects of the condition directly, as do symptoms, signs, and tests, but rather measures the impact of the condition on day-to-day life. Many generic health status measures operate on the functional level, but most of them use reported function rather than direct testing of performance.

Care needs to be exercised with measures that utilize function tests. A test that measures, for example, a patient's ability to walk a specified distance measures just that: the ability of a patient to walk a specified distance. This point may seem quite obvious but is often overlooked. Investigators often use function tests to measure some underlying disease state. For example, if arthritis limits the ability to walk, does a test of a person's ability to walk measure arthritis? To answer "yes" involves a leap of faith (and is also a logical fallacy). This leap can be made but should only be made in the presence of a strong conceptual model. Consider the following as an example of the type of mistake that this approach could allow. An investigator attempts to measure the relationship between an intervention and arthritis, using walking distance as a function test. The intervention is exercise. The experimental group increases its fitness level as a result of the exercise and, therefore, walks further, although the arthritis is unchanged. Increased scores on the function test, driven by changes in fitness levels, are then falsely interpreted as improvements in arthritis.

Each type of test has different shortcomings and will tap a different domain of the impact of the condition on the patient. Many domains can be measured by each of the different methods. For example, a measure of health could be a function test (like activities of daily living [ADL]) or a symptom reported by a patient (self-reported health).

Rheumatoid arthritis can provide an example of the hierarchy of measure that may be involved. Spiegel and her colleagues (1986) examined some of the available condition-specific tests for rheumatoid arthritis to explore which domains each measure covered. First, symptoms are reported by the patient: morning stiffness and pain. Next, signs can be discovered on physical examination: tenderness, swelling of joints, and joint deformity. Tests are available, such as x-rays and laboratory tests for the presence of an inflammatory disorder. A series of performance tests is available, notably a grip test and a walk time test. Finally, generic health status measures such as ADLs can measure functional status. Which is the correct test to use?

Rheumatoid arthritis is a chronic, symmetrical arthritis affecting synovial lining of joints. Initially, the patient typically experiences swelling and tenderness of affected joints, followed by pain and stiffness. Eventually, the range of motion of the joints may become limited, joints may become deformed, and cysts may form. Other problems associated with rheumatoid arthritis include malaise and anemia. Although other complications are much less common, rheumatoid arthritis can affect almost every organ system, including the heart and lungs. This is an example of a disease primarily associated with the musculoskeletal system having complications in many different systems (which argues for the inclusion of a generic health status measure along with a condition-specific measure).

There is no cure for rheumatoid arthritis. Interventions include exercises and splints for sleeping to increase range of motion (also surgery in extreme cases). Symptomatic pharmacologic therapy can reduce inflammation. Rheumatoid arthritis is rarely fatal, but pain, suffering, and impairment can be extreme. Up to 15% of patients become fully incapacitated (Fishman, 1985).

With this background, the question of which test to use can be asked again. Which measure is appropriate depends entirely on the research question. Measures that address treatment for an acute exacerbation may be very different from those that address performance. Acute measures concentrate on tests of the effects of inflammatory response, such as joint counts and sedimentation rates. Investigators using function tests, like walk time and grip strength, to detect acute events must consider that they are strongly related to joint deformity. Regardless of a person's acute status, extensive joint deformity may dramatically impair performance. In contrast, clinical estimates of disease activity and pain by physicians and patients (signs and symptoms) appear to be strongly related to disease activity but not as strongly to functional status. Global functioning may be affected by a person's mental state. Depressed or discouraged patients may find themselves less able to cope with social roles at the same level of disease activity as those unimpaired by such feelings. The choice of an appropriate outcome measure for rheumatoid arthritis depends entirely on the expected impact of the intervention and knowledge of the relationship of the measure to other clinically significant factors.

When selecting a particular condition-specific measure, the investigator should have built a conceptual model to facilitate the identification of important domains. In this rheumatoid arthritis example, it is necessary to understand the natural history of the disease and the expected impact of the intervention prior to the selection of the condition-specific measure. The bottom line is that in order to select an appropriate condition-specific measure, investigators must know what they wish to measure.

The Role of Condition-Specific versus Generic Measures

Generic and condition-specific measures can complement each other. The domains measured by condition-specific measures may resemble those addressed by generic measures, but they are treated differently. When an investigator selects a condition-specific measure, the reason is typically to measure domains more deeply than they are measured by generic measures. The cataract eye surgery study mentioned earlier provides an example of this goal (Damiano et al., 1995). If it is decided to use both condition-specific and generic measures, the investigator should be clear as to why both are being included in the study. Often, generic measures are used as a safety net; they are designed to capture unexpected results of the intervention. This is not generally a wise strategy because it can lead to statistical trolling: casting a wide net without an underlying model in the hopes that something will prove interesting in retrospect. This strategy is often used early on in the research of a new treatment.

Typical statistical measures, such as t-tests, are designed to test hypotheses. If a 95% significance level is used to test hypotheses, then Type I errors (rejecting the null hypothesis when the null hypothesis is true) will occur 5% of the time. Therefore, in 20 tests, 1 would be expected to be significant simply due to chance. Simply throwing a battery of tests at a problem, without any theory, can lead to false conclusions.

Instead, generic measures should be incorporated to test specific hypotheses. An intervention's primary impact may be in one domain, but the intervention may also be expected to have secondary impacts in several different domains. For example, knee surgery might affect not just mobility but could potentially also affect other domains, such as mental health (if increased mobility reduced depression caused by isolation).

Another reason for incorporating generic measures into a study is that overall health, as measured by generic health measures, may differentially affect the intervention's impact on the main (condition-specific) outcome measure. Consider, for example, back surgery as an intervention for patients with back pain. The purpose of the intervention is to decrease pain. A condition-specific outcome measure, such as the Roland Low Back Pain Rating Scale (Roland & Morris, 1983), could be used to measure the levels of pain both before and after the intervention. The success of the intervention may depend on overall health status. People suffering from a multitude of ailments may not gain much relief from the surgery, even if the surgery worked perfectly. Such a result does not mean the intervention was a failure; rather, it means the success of the surgery depends on overall health status. A condition-specific measure can convey the result that the surgery worked, which is necessary information for the narrow evaluation of the surgery. A generic measure could reveal that, for some patients, the surgery had no positive impact on the overall well-being of the patient. The latter information is necessary for evaluating, for example, the cost-effectiveness of a treatment, or it could be used in targeting a treatment toward populations likely to gain benefit from the treatment.

Choosing a Measure

Selecting the best condition-specific health status measure for a study can be difficult. Investigators can either create a new measure or use an already developed measure. Despite the appeal of a customized measure, the work involved is substantial, and the acceptance of the results of the study may hinge on the acceptance of the measure. Pioneering investigators must first provide strong and convincing evidence that their measure is reliable, internally consistent, and valid before even beginning to discuss the substantive results of the study. Further, the results of the study with the new measure will be hard to compare with those from any previous study. These drawbacks, combined with the time and cost associated with the development of a new measure, argue strongly against it unless no available measures are acceptable.

The better option is to choose a condition-specific measure developed and validated by other investigators. For many conditions, there are a multitude of condition-specific measures (e.g., for the measurement of arthritis, at least five standard condition-specific outcome measures are available; Patrick & Deyo, 1989).

The selection of a particular condition-specific measure from the measures available should be guided by statistical, theoretical, and practical criteria. Statistically, the investigator should seek measures that are reliable, valid, unbiased, precise in the range where effects are expected, and easy to implement (Kessler & Mroczek, 1995). An extended discussion of these issues is available in Chapter 9.

Theoretically, the measure should cover the domains of greatest interest. The determination of the domains must be driven by a theoretical model of the disease or condition and how it will interact with the treatment.

Practical considerations should be taken into account. The mode of administration of the measure needs to be consistent with the overall design of the study. For example, it would be improper to have study participants self-administer a measure designed for use in a telephone survey. Measures that have been used previously in similar studies should be given preference over infrequently used or new measures. Widely used measures will facilitate comparisons of the results of the study with those of previous studies.

The investigator should also consider the distribution of expected scores in the study population. Scales that fail to adequately distinguish between the population should be avoided. If there is a floor or ceiling effect, the study will not yield any results, regardless of the effectiveness of the intervention. For example, if the study population consists of frail older adults, avoid as much as possible measures designed for healthy populations. A different, but equally important shortcoming of a measure is when all the respondents bunch in the middle of the scale. In this case, again, shortcomings in the measure may prevent successful measurement of an intervention. Measures selected should be capable of distinguishing between participants in the intervention.

Some measures require the use of complicated scoring algorithms. Some are also bulky or complicated. All other things equal, simpler and shorter is better.

The time frame of measures also varies. For example, the SF-36 asks about the previous 4 weeks. Other measures may ask about the previous 6 months. Some may ask about right now. A measure should be selected with a time frame appropriate for the intervention and condition.

It is also worth considering how the results of the study will be analyzed. The method of analysis should be established prior to the beginning of the study. This allows the investigator to select appropriate statistical tests and thereby to conduct a power analysis and determine sample size.

CONCLUSION

The proper selection of the outcomes measure is a key to any successful outcomes study. The best approach to picking a measure is first to acquire an understanding of the natural history of the condition, then develop a theory of how the intervention will interact with the condition. This will allow for the discovery of the domains where the intervention is expected to have impact.

Condition-specific measures are focused, precise measures that are able to delve deeply into the domains of greatest interest. Condition-specific measures should be teamed with appropriate generic measures so that the intervention can be evaluated not just for its narrow impact on the condition but also for its impact on overall health across a multitude of domains.

Condition-specific measures can play a central role in assessing the outcomes of care. They are best seen as complements to, rather than substitutes for, generic measures. Some condition-specific measures come directly from clinical practice. Others must be created. Care must be exercised not to place undue confidence in the reliability of measures derived directly from practice.

REFERENCES

Barry, M., Fowler, F., O'Leary, M., Bruskewitz, R., Holtgrewe, L., Mebust, W., & The Measurement Committee of the American Urological Association (1995). Measuring disease-specific health status in men with benign prostatic hyperplasia. *Medical Care, 33*(S4), AS145–AS155.

Bergner, M., Bobbitt, R., Kressel, S., Pollard, W., Gilson, B., & Morris, J. (1976). The Sickness Impact Profile: Conceptual formulation and methodological development of a health status index. *International Journal of Health Services, 6,* 393.

Berlowitz, D.R., Ash, A.S., Hickey, E.C., Friedman, R.H., Kader, B., & Moskowitz, M.A. (in press). Outcomes of hypertension care: Simple measures are not that simple. *Medical Care.*

Bombardier, C., Melfi, C., Paul, J., Green, R., Hawker, G., Wright, J., & Coyte, P. (1995). Comparison of a generic and a disease specific measure of pain and physical function after knee replacement surgery. *Medical Care, 33*(S4), AS131–AS144.

Damiano, A., Steinberg, E., Cassard, S., Bass, E., Diener-West, M., Legro, M., Tielsch, J., Schein, O., Javitt, J., & Kolb, M. (1995). Comparison of generic versus disease specific measures of functional impairment in patients with cataract. *Medical Care, 33*(S4), AS120–AS130.

Elmore, J., Wells, C., Lee, C., Howard, D., & Feinstein, A. (1994). Variability in radiologists' interpretations of mammograms. *New England Journal of Medicine, 331*(22), 1,493–1,499.

Feinstein, A.R. (1977). *Clinical biostatistics*. St. Louis: Mosby.

Fishman, R.A. (1985). Normal-pressure hydrocephalus and arthritis. *New England Journal of Medicine, 312*(19), 1,255–1,256.

Guyatt, G.H., Feeny, D.H., & Patrick, D.L. (1993). Measuring health-related quality of life. *Annals of Internal Medicine, 118*, 622–629.

Idler, E.L., & Kasl, S. (1991). Health perceptions and survival: Do global evaluations of health status really predict mortality? *Journal of Gerontology, 46*(2), S55–S65.

Kazis, L.E., Anderson, J.J., & Meenan, R.F. (1989). Effect sizes for interpreting changes in health status. *Medical Care, 27*(3 suppl.), S178–S189.

Kessler, R., & Mroczek, D. (1995). Measuring the effects of medical interventions. *Medical Care, 33*(S4), AS109–AS119.

Kjerulff, K., & Langenberg, P. (1995). A comparison of alternative ways of measuring fatigue among patients having hysterectomy. *Medical Care, 33*(S4), AS156–AS163.

Koos, E.L. (1954). *The health of Regionville*. New York: Columbia University Press.

McNair, D., Lorr, M., & Droppleman, L. (1971). *EITS Manual of the Profile of Mood States*. San Diego: Education and Industrial Testing Service.

Meredith, L.S., & Siu, A.L. (1995). Variation and quality of self-report health data: Asian and Pacific Islanders compared with other ethnic groups. *Medical Care, 33*(11), 1,120–1,131.

Patrick, D.L., & Deyo, R.A. (1989). Generic and disease-specific measures in assessing health status and quality of life. *Medical Care, 27*(3), S217–S232.

Roland M., & Morris, R. (1983). A study of the natural history of back pain, Part I: Development of a reliable and sensitive measure of disability in low-back pain. *Spine, 8*(2), 141–150.

Sherbourne, C., & Meredith, L. (1992). Quality of self-report data: A comparison of older and younger chronically ill patients. *Journal of Gerontology, 47*(4), S204–S211.

Spiegel, J.S., Paulus, H., Ward, N., Spiegel, T., Leake, B., & Kane, R. (1986). What are we measuring? An examination of self-reported functional status measures. *Arthritis and Rheumatism, 31*(6), 721–728.

Steinberg, E., Tielsch, J., Schein, O., Javitt, J., Sharkey, D., Cassard, S., Legro, M., Diener-West, M., Bass, E., & Damiano, A. (1994). The VF-14: An index of functional impairment in cataract patients. *Arch Ophthalomol*, 112: 630.

Stewart, A., Hays, R., & Ware J. (1988). The MOS short-form general health survey: Reliability and validity in a patient population. *Medical Care, 26*, 724.

Temkin, N.R., Dikmen, S., Machamer, J., & McLean, A. (1989). General versus disease-specific measures: Further work on the sickness impact profile for head injury. *Medical Care, 27*(3), S44–S53.

Ware, J.E. Jr., & Sherbourne, C.D. (1992). The MOS 36-item short-form health survey (SF-36). I. Conceptual framework and item selection. *Medical Care, 30*(6), 473–483.

Zborowski, M. (1952). Cultural components in response to pain. *Journal of Social Issues, 8*, 16–30.

4

Satisfaction

Matthew Maciejewski
Jacalyn Kawiecki
Todd Rockwood

CHAPTER OUTLINE

- What Is Satisfaction?
- How Do Marketing Models Relate to Patient Satisfaction?
- The Clinical Model of Satisfaction: Where To Begin?
- Why Measure Satisfaction?
- How Can Satisfaction Be Measured?
- What Are the Critical Methodological Issues?
- Are Existing Satisfaction Measures Available for Researchers?
- What Can Be Expected from Future Measures?

The legitimacy of patient satisfaction as an outcome measure of health care has grown considerably over the past decade. Patient satisfaction has been used for a variety of purposes in different settings. Satisfaction is considered an indicator of quality of care. Satisfaction is also being used to assess the performance of health care delivery at multiple levels—organizational (hospital, clinic, etc.), unit (surgical, laboratory, radiology, etc.), and individual (physician, nurses, etc.). Patient satisfaction is also being used to evaluate and develop patient care models (such as patient-centered care models put forth by the Picker–Commonwealth Institute). In the new era of health care, where quality assurance, continuous quality improvement (CQI), total quality management (TQM), and cost effectiveness are actively pursued, patient satisfaction assumes even more importance (Kennedy, 1996). As the paradigm for health care shifts toward a marketplace model, exemplified by managed care, consumer satisfaction becomes the outcome with economic implications. Satisfaction is an outcome of care that directly reflects consumers' opinions and, hence, their likelihood to stay enrolled in a managed care plan or to use a specific care provider. Satisfaction thus has marketing as well as quality implications.

The interest in patient satisfaction for marketing and quality assurance purposes has outpaced advances in its conceptualization and measurement (Carey & Seibert, 1993). Surveys are often done without careful consideration of what is being measured and the limitations in the results obtained. The major challenge in the development of satisfaction measures is how to capture the patient's perspective in terms that are at once meaningful to patients, and which lend themselves to aggregation and scaling. If survey questions cannot be summed to obtain subscales or an overall score, it is difficult to make summary statements comparing satisfaction across clinical settings. Empirical research on patient satisfaction has demonstrated a number of problems, including:

- a lack of accepted conceptual or theoretical model of the determinants of patient satisfaction
- methodological dilemmas and a lack of standardized approaches to assess patient satisfaction
- a paucity of studies that compare care across clinical settings
- a lack of consensus within the medical profession on what role patient satisfaction should play (Arahony & Strasser, 1993)

This chapter explores these issues and provides a framework that will motivate investigators to include patient satisfaction in their assessments of outcomes.

WHAT IS SATISFACTION?

Any clinician interested in measuring patient satisfaction first must ask several questions: How do the consumers (patients) think about satisfaction? How do they know they are satisfied? What criteria do they use to determine their satisfaction? The answers to these deceptively simple questions are based on one's conceptual model of patient satisfaction.

Assessing patient satisfaction requires the consideration of two conceptual aspects: (1) a theoretically derived definition of the concept, and (2) a methodological definition that allows its operationalization. The first step explicates the role for the concept and how it relates to other concepts (e.g., the relationship of patient satisfaction and health status). A theoretical model gives context to the main construct—satisfaction—in relation to the causes and effects of outcomes in a clinical experience. A good model clearly links satisfaction in a hierarchy or chain of causation. For example, one might posit that satisfaction is based upon patient–physician interaction, and compliance is based upon the level of satisfaction the patient comes away with. Patient satisfaction in this model can also be illustrated as:

Interaction ——▶ Satisfaction ——▶ Compliance

The second step moves the concept from abstraction to measurement in empirical research. The importance of this step cannot be overstated, because two different people may come up with two different definitions of satisfaction when working with the same fundamental concept. Some researchers may interpret patient satisfaction to be a function of a physician's bedside manner, while others believe it to be a function of the cost of care. As in many intellectual endeavors, where one stands depends critically on where one sits. While satisfaction has been repeatedly measured and used to assess the quality of care, little of this work has attempted to systematically address these fundamental issues.

Definitions of *patient satisfaction* are scarce, but the following are pertinent:

- *Patient satisfaction* is a patient's (affective or emotional) response to his or her (cognitive or knowledge-based) evaluation of the health care provider's performance (perceived quality) during a health care consumption experience (Ross et al., 1987).

- *Patient satisfaction* is a health care recipient's reaction to salient aspects of his or her service experience (Pascoe, 1983).

These two definitions of satisfaction share similar components: (1) satisfaction is a patient's emotional or cognitive evaluation of a health care provider's performance, and (2) the evaluation is based upon relevant aspects of the experience. These conceptual models are based on work that has started to converge from two distinct fields—marketing research and clinical practice. Marketing theories posit that satisfaction is based on the characteristics of the good, as well as the gestalt in which the good or service is obtained. Models motivated by clinical practice often focus on technical competency and the interpersonal aspects of care as the major determinants of patient satisfaction.

Information asymmetry causes evaluations of quality in a clinical setting to be more complicated than assessments of, for example, the quality of a stereo. Stereos can be judged from objective sources of information such as *Consumer Reports*, prior experience with stereos, and comparative shopping and testing of various brands. Satisfaction with a clinical experience is necessarily subjective. Satisfaction is closer to outcomes like pain and depression than to functioning because it relies heavily on subjective evaluation and interpretation.

Patient satisfaction can address many aspects of care. The dimensions of patient satisfaction that are most frequently assessed include the interpersonal aspects of care, technical quality of care, accessibility and availability of care, continuity of care, patient convenience, physical setting, financial considerations, efficacy, communication, respect, time spent, and concern (Ware, Davies-Avery, & Stewart, 1978; Ware et al., 1983).

Interpersonal Aspects of Care

The way patients feel about those caring for them is essential. Patients want their caregivers to care. Interpersonal dimensions include such aspects as the concern the provider seems to feel about the patient as a person as well as a case, the provider's respect shown for the patient, and the time spent with the patient. In general, patients want to be recognized as individuals. They want their examinations to be thorough. They may have to wait to see a physician, but, once they are seen, the visit should take as long as necessary. Providers need to give the patient their full attention and not be distracted by other demands.

The extent and accuracy of communication between physicians and patients is the most frequently studied aspect of medical care. Patient satisfaction is correlated to self-reports and independent ratings of both the amount and the clarity of the information given by the physician (Housten & Pasanen, 1972) and, thus, may be a useful marker of the quality of physician–patient communication (Lochman, 1983). The aspect of care in which patients are least satisfied is often physician communication.

Patient satisfaction is found to be higher if the sociodemographic characteristics of the physician are similar to those of the patient, if patients are allowed to express themselves when giving their medical history, and if the physician is informative and shares control during the conclusion of the interview (Cleary & McNeil, 1988). Generally, in those studies where satisfaction with communication of health care information is measured, this variable tended to be one of the most important elements of overall satisfaction (Cleary & McNeil, 1988; Doering, 1983).

Accessibility, Availability, and Convenience of Care

This dimension of care includes waiting time to get an appointment and waiting time in the office. Other physical problems may involve the location of services, the time the offices are open, and the ease of reaching them. Aspects of access extend beyond physical boundaries. They address how easily help can be obtained in an emergency, whether there is direct access to specialists (or sophisticated tests), and whether some type of prior approval is needed. Convenience is closely linked to access. The times services are available and the ease of reaching them are central issues. Scheduling that accommodates the patients' needs can prove an important element.

Continuity of Care

Continuity can refer to seeing the same provider or to the sense that information is transferred from one episode of care to another or from one provider to another. For example, primary care referrals to specialists involve the transfer of information both before and after the consultation. In group practices, patients may not always see the same physician, but they want to sense that whoever is caring for them knows their history and hopefully something about them as people. Repeatedly being asked the same questions as if starting anew each time can be a frustrating experience. A central aspect of this dimension is the patients' sense that the care system knows them and their problems.

Physical Setting

Patients may express dissatisfaction with the actual arrangement of the care setting in terms of its shabbiness or its overall design. It may not be accessible to the disabled. It may be difficult to find one's way, especially if there is poor signage. The furniture may not be comfortable. Parking may be a problem, or the walk from the parking facility to the clinic may be overly taxing.

Technical Quality of Care

The quality of medical care is determined primarily by the technical competence of the provider for many health care professionals. However, assessing technical quality is complicated and difficult for patients in the evaluation of their care. Several studies have found that perceived competence is related to patient satisfaction (Pascoe, 1983), but there have been few studies of whether satisfaction is related to an independent rating of technical performance (Shortell et al., 1977). Overall, the research indicates that satisfaction is related to perceptions of technical skills, intelligence, and qualifications, but perceived interpersonal and communication skills generally account for more of the variation in patient satisfaction (Cleary & McNeil, 1988).

Efficacy

Efficacy refers to the helpfulness of medical providers in improving or maintaining health (Marquis, Davies, & Ware, 1983). It is closely linked to discussion about patients' abilities to judge the technical aspects of care. Patient beliefs in the efficacy of the treatment can be central to its effectiveness. Occasionally, conflicts develop when patients insist on care that is not deemed to be scientifically supported. Patient confidence can be influenced by the style of care as well as its science. In general, most explorations of patient satisfaction do not ask patients to comment directly on their impressions about the efficacy of care per se, although the patients may be asked such things as whether they would opt for the same experience or how they feel about the outcomes achieved.

Financial Considerations

The cost of care can affect satisfaction. Both the direct costs levied and the ways they are collected can influence patients' feelings about their care. Because insurance plays a central role, the net costs may be different from the charges. The way billing information is transmitted and the stringency of demands for payment can color one's feelings about the care received.

HOW DO MARKETING MODELS RELATE TO PATIENT SATISFACTION?

Well-developed theories of satisfaction exist in the marketing and social psychology literature, but the links between this work and health services research have been limited (Churchill & Suprenant, 1982; Tse, Franco, & Wilton, 1990). Satisfaction is a multidimensional, dynamic construct that can vary across time and individuals (Strasser, Arahony, & Greenberger, 1993). Evaluations of satisfaction have both emotional and cognitive components. As stated earlier, satisfaction is an attitudinal response to value judgments that patients make about their clinical encounters. Patients arrive at their judgments by comparing their expectations with the actual performance of their clinical encounter. Expectations, in turn, are based on perceptions of previous experiences. Expectations play a critical role in these theories by providing the baseline or basis of comparison. These models assume that individuals have prior experience on which to rationally form expectations. If patients have no prior experience, they must form expectations from other sources of information. Alternative sources are opinions of significant others, information from pamphlets, videos, and physician advice.

Health care differs from typical marketing situations because physicians can act as agents for patients. Whereas consumers do not use a stereo or grocery consultant to help them elicit their preferences and then translate expectations into consumption, physicians may take on this agency role, especially in cases of elective surgery. Basing expectations of performance partly on a physician's expert opinion may influence patient's evaluations of care. If physicians influence expectations when patients do not have previous experience, satisfaction and compliance behavior may become more predictable. At the same time, more discriminating measures of patient satisfaction may be derived.

THE CLINICAL MODEL OF SATISFACTION: WHERE TO BEGIN?

Finding the right measure of satisfaction requires careful consideration of one's own conceptual model of satisfaction and that implicit in the measure under consideration. No comprehensive formulation is available, but some observations seem to pertain:

- Satisfaction is a distinct outcome of care, although it is closely related to health status outcomes (Kane, Maciejewski, & Finch, in press).
- Satisfaction is derived from many sources, including the gestalt of the health care episode and the particular dimensions of care salient to the patient.
- Satisfaction is a subjective evaluation (either emotional or cognitive) that may be influenced by the opinions of others or based on previous experience.
- The dimensions of care covered in a satisfaction measure should be based on the investigator's conception of satisfaction.

This dependence entirely on patient evaluation has led to difficulties in clearly conceptualizing and operationalizing satisfaction and to clinician reluctance to act on or be judged on the basis of patient satisfaction. The subjective nature of patient satisfaction allows for confounding results. For example, two patients with the same baseline pre- and post-intervention health status and outcome may diverge in satisfaction with care. Assuming their demographic characteristics are the same, the source of variation may be life experience or outlook. This result would not support a model that posited that satisfaction is based upon outcome. Clinicians are justifiably frustrated by such findings. Attention must be given to assessment of the specific dimensions or aspects of care thought to be relevant to patients.

While much research remains to be done to clarify the theoretical and conceptual foundations of patient satisfaction, interest in this aspect of outcomes research will not wait for the development of the satisfaction gold standard. Thoughtful consideration of pitfalls can explicate, if not eliminate, the possible limitations of previous research. As with all outcome measures, one must consider the scaling and weighting of responses in patient satisfaction surveys. (Chapter 9 on measurement provides a more detailed summary of how to address these issues.)

WHY MEASURE SATISFACTION?

Donabedian states that achieving and producing health and satisfaction, as defined for its individual members by a particular society or subculture, is the ultimate validator of the quality of care (Donabedian, 1966). This prophetic statement is coming true as patient satisfaction and outcomes are being used as indicators of quality through report cards, clinical guidelines, and satisfaction surveys. Patient satisfaction is being used for a variety of purposes, and discriminating purchasers must understand the goals that satisfaction information serves in different contexts. Marketing materials by health plans and hospitals invariably include some mention of how highly consumers value their services. If all providers in an area indicate that their patients are highly satisfied, price becomes the only factor that differentiates them. This not uncommon situation can be improved upon by using satisfaction surveys that discriminate better across different dimensions of providers. Although there are as many arguments concerning why satisfaction measurement should be used as there are people who use it, some of the most frequently cited reasons are (Arahony & Strasser, 1993).

- **Patients can play an important role in defining how health care is delivered.** Models of such patient-centered care were in part developed based on the assessment of patient satisfaction (University Hospital Consortium, 1995).
- **Patients can play an important role in defining quality care by determining what values should be associated with different outcomes.** While they may not have the necessary knowledge to assess the technical aspect of the care they receive, patients appreciate its importance. (Cleary & McNeil, 1988).
- **The quality of physicians' interpersonal skills influences patient outcomes.** The effects of physician communication skills on patients' adherence to medical regimes are mediated by patient satisfaction and recall (Bartlett et al., 1984). Medical/nursing and other staffs' attitudes toward patients and physician–patient communication can reduce the use of pain medication, shorten lengths of stay, and improve patient compliance (Press, Ganey, & Malone, 1990).

- **Satisfaction can affect outcomes through a placebo effect, which in some instances, has been shown to contribute to up to one-third of the actual healing process** (Press et al., 1990).
- **As medical care increasingly becomes a consumer good, patient (customer) satisfaction becomes more salient.** In the context of managed care, satisfaction determines continued enrollment (Arahony & Strasser, 1993).

Satisfaction has been tied to many aspects of the health care universe: behavior (plan, institution, provider, patient), communication, referrals, recidivism, and other factors, but it has not been without its share of problems. Patient satisfaction is perhaps the most important evaluative outcome in a patient's health care experience. It affects many things, including future behavioral intentions, word-of-mouth communications, and referrals (John, 1992). Prior satisfaction with the health care system in general and with the same hospital when applicable can be a significant influence on patient evaluations of current hospital experiences (John, 1992). Levels of patient satisfaction and compliance are presumed to affect other subsequent outcomes, such as patient's health status, continuity of care, and the frequency and length of hospitalization (Lochman, 1983).

HOW CAN SATISFACTION BE MEASURED?

Those who criticize attempts to measure patient satisfaction often point to the problems inherent in measuring any amorphous concept such as satisfaction or quality. In the prior section, we addressed this criticism by illustrating the specific, tangible aspects of medical encounters that one can measure. In this section, we focus on the challenge of measurement. Some of the issues raised by critics can be partially, if not completely, controlled through careful design, survey development, and measurement method.

The results of satisfaction evaluations depend heavily on the selected measurement method (e.g., surveys, focus groups) (Ware & Hays, 1988; Ross, Steward, & Sinacore, 1995). In addition, different measures capture various dimensions of satisfaction, since patients may express satisfaction with different aspects of care. Patients may feel satisfied with a physician's affective behavior (humaneness or bedside manner), but feel dissatisfied with the thoroughness or informativeness of the provider. These and other issues need to be addressed in a series of questions to answer the question of how to measure satisfaction.

Contrasting opinions have been expressed regarding patient evaluation of care and appropriate measures of satisfaction. Although few satisfaction measures exist, comparative analyses of measures to validate these measures are rare.

Comparisons of global and specific satisfaction measures need to be done, as well as comparisons of alternative measures of the same general type.

Global measures that address satisfaction with overall care are used more often than specific encounter measures, but overall global measures are probably less useful in identifying problem areas or assessing quality of care because they do not discriminate as well. It is often difficult to make sense of empirical findings or explain discrepancies across satisfaction studies because some researchers measure satisfaction before they consider the theoretical meaning or psychometric properties of satisfaction measures (Locker & Dunt, 1978). Often, researchers have not differentiated the type of satisfaction measured (Cleary & McNeil, 1988).

Issues in measurement of patient satisfaction are similar to those for generic and specific health status measures. There is often a tradeoff between the number of aspects and depth of coverage of those aspects in the measurement of patient satisfaction. Researchers must ask themselves how specific they want to get when assessing satisfaction, because global measures and measures for specific medical encounters will have a different overall focus in evaluating satisfaction. The choice of measure(s) will depend upon the outcome sought by the researcher.

Patients' judgments about the quality of their care are closely linked to their satisfaction with that care. Previous research has indicated that outcomes lead to satisfaction (Hall, Milburn, & Epstein, 1993), but both terms need careful attention. *Outcomes* can be expressed in two ways: outcome at follow-up (absolute value) or outcome change from baseline (relative value) (Aseltine et al., 1995).

WHAT ARE THE CRITICAL METHODOLOGICAL ISSUES?

All of the standard social research methods can be used to measure satisfaction: archival, ethnographic, focus groups, and survey research.[1] The last two methods are the most common formats used to collect data on patient satisfaction. However, open-ended (ethnographic) interviews with patients can provide a rich understanding of the dynamics of the health care provision process from a patient's point of view. This type of format tends not to constrain the focus of discussion on the issues considered significant by the interviewer only. Focus groups have also been utilized to assess satisfaction. They have several advantages, but results from these discussions cannot be generalized beyond the sample studied. Focus groups can provide qualitative, as well as quantitative, data; they permit detailed exploration of specific events and present an opportunity for spontaneous information to emerge.

Survey Research

Survey administration is the most common method to assess satisfaction. The advantage of survey research over other methods hinges upon several factors. If conducted properly, a survey allows a sample of a population to be studied and the findings can be generalized to an entire population. A survey relies on the standardization of measurement whereby all respondents are presented with the same stimuli (questions) and constrained to respond in a uniform manner (closed response categories). This standardization avoids the introduction of sources of bias possible in other formats. Readers are referred to Sudman and Bradburn (1974) for a comprehensive discussion of survey research.

Administration and Sampling

Selecting which mode to use to administer a survey—telephone, face-to-face, or self-administered (often by mail)—is usually driven by two factors: cost and the relative convenience of one mode over another. The cost of different administration modes will depend primarily on the total number of respondents and time required for each survey. The time required for each survey is a function of the length and complexity of the survey. Most satisfaction research is based on the telephone and mail modes of administration. The telphone mode allows for quicker feedback and permits some interactions for explanations and clarifications of questions. It is, however, more susceptible to the problem of social desirability.

Social desirability is the tendency of respondents to offer answers that are consistent with values the respondent believes to be held by the interviewer (Groves, 1989; Groves, et al., 1988; Locander, Sudman & Bradburn, 1976). This social influence, which pressures the respondent to provide a response that is in line with normative expectations or self-enhancing presentation, is influenced both by the mode of survey administration as well as the substantive content of the question. As noted above, the mail mode of survey administration is less susceptible to social desirability than the telephone or face-to-face modes of administration.

Respondents are often unwilling to disclose what they really think and instead provide normative responses (i.e., that they are satisfied). This positive response bias is reflected in the overwhelming high approval ratings that are continually found in almost all satisfaction surveys (Carr-Hill, 1992). The mode of survey administration influences this effect (Aquilino, 1994; Dillman et al., 1996). Mailed surveys, while not immune to the influence of social desirability, are less susceptible than both the telephone and face-to-face modes (de Leeuw, 1992; Dillman et al., 1996).

Aside from selecting the mail mode, there are two primary techniques for dealing with social desirability: confidentiality guarantees and question structure. Setting up means to ensure confidentiality and conveying this information to respondents has been demonstrated to reduce error due to social desirability, but overemphasizing such guarantees can produce a reverse effect (Singer, Von

Thurn, & Miller, 1995). (See works such as Dillman [1978] and Salant & Dillman [1994] for examples of confidentiality wording as well as mechanisms to ensure the confidentiality of the respondent.)

Regardless of the mode used to administer a survey, poor response rates are a persistent problem. The problem usually does not lie with the sampling frame.[2] While there are multiple ways of calculating response rates (Groves, 1989), the response rate is typically calculated as follows:

Response rate = Number of completed surveys/Number of surveys distributed.[3]

Although there is no set standard for what constitutes an acceptable response rate, significant response error can be introduced when the response rate is low (Groves, 1989). Convention has indicated a response rate below 60% raises serious concern regarding error due to non-response[4] and suggests that the data should not be used. With planning and commitment, including using techniques such as the Total Design Method (Dillman, 1978; Salant & Dillman, 1994), an acceptable response rate can be achieved.

Any time a sample of a population is surveyed and the response rate is not 100%, the possibility of sampling error is introduced. Sampling error is an error of nonobservation, based on surveying a sample of a population rather than the entire population. From any given population, a number of samples could be drawn, and a different sample could produce a different distribution of the characteristic in the population. The sampling error estimates the range that the distribution of the characteristic could have within the population. (See Groves [1989] for a discussion of the implications of sampling error for survey research; see Hansen, Hurwitz, & Madow [1953]), Kish [1965], and Wolter [1985] for a discussion of the estimation of survey research.) While there are means of calculating the actual sampling error, as a rule of thumb, the following is the margin of error associated with typical sample size: n = 100 +/- 10%, n = 500 +/- 5%, n = 1,000 +/- 3%, n = 2,000 +/- 2%. This range of error does not mean that the "true value" of response falls within that range. It refers only to sampling error and has no consideration of measurement error, which can change the distribution of response by 20% or more (Schuman & Presser, 1981).

Measurement Error

Measurement error is of great concern. Simply changing the wording in a question (e.g., from "welfare" to "support for families and children in need") can change the response significantly (Schuman et al., 1981). Satisfaction research is susceptible to all four of the main sources of measurement error: interviewers, respondents, questionnaires, and mode of administration (Groves, 1989). While there is no means of completely overcoming measurement error, good question development and questionnaire layout can help in reducing its impact.

Interviewers

Interviewers in the telephone and face-to-face mode of administration can influence response in a number of ways. (See Groves [1989] for a review.) Two factors seem particularly relevant to satisfaction research. First, if the interviewer is seen by the respondent as representing the sponsoring agency (such as hospital, clinic, health plan, etc.), then respondents are much less likely to be as forthcoming in their responses (Groves et al., 1988; Schuman & Presser, 1981). Second are both inter-interviewer as well as intra-interviewer (across participants) differences in conducting interviews (Groves et al., 1988; Schuman & Presser, 1981). Careful training and supervision, along with regular monitoring, are essential.

Respondents

Measurement error associated with respondents can be manifested in a number of ways. In satisfaction research, three fundamental characteristics of respondents have been identified as primary areas of concern. First is respondent expertise. For many aspects of health care, patients lack the expertise or technical knowledge to provide an informed evaluation of that part of the encounter. Contrasting opinions have been expressed regarding patient evaluations of care. Although patients have been shown to be able to distinguish various aspects of care (Ware et al., 1983), patients' abilities to evaluate technical quality have been questioned (DiMatteo & Hays, 1980). Older patients and patients of low socioeconomic status are less able to differentiate technical ability and affective behavior than are younger patients and patients of higher socioeconomic status (DiMatteo & Hays, 1980). Information derived from patients can be used to assess other aspects of care delivered, patient functioning, and symptoms (Davies & Ware, 1988; Ware et al., 1983). One direct reflection of patient dissatisfaction may be changing care providers (Marquis et al., 1983; Wersinger & Sorenson, 1982).

The second and third aspects are closely related: acquiescence and social desirability. *Acquiescence* is the tendency of the respondent to agree with a statement (Schuman & Presser, 1981). In satisfaction research, this has been linked to *response-set bias* (Ware & Hays, 1988), the tendency of respondents, when presented with a list of items, to pick one particular response category and answer all questions on the list with that response. The acquiescence problem can be addressed through the design of questions and instruments. Rather than using long lists of items that share the same set of response categories, breaking these lists up into smaller groups can reduce acquiescent responses. Questions should not all be written in a particular direction (usually positive). It is better to place both positively and negatively worded items into a single, balanced scale. This technique, however, may reduce the internal consistency of the scale (Ross et al., 1995).

The final aspect dealing with respondents addresses how they formulate their responses (Schwarz & Sudman, 1996). Satisfaction ratings appear to be influenced by the timing of administration (Ley, Kinsey, & Atherton, 1976). Patients asked about their satisfaction with a facility before seeing a physician may give different responses if asked the same questions after seeing a physician. The intervening experience of the physician encounter may have a moderating effect even though judgments of a facility should be distinct from judgments of physician encounters. Another problem is the telescoping of events (i.e., either bringing things from the past forward in time or pushing things backward in time) (Baddeley, 1979; Loftus et al., 1990). These problems can be overcome by tying the response to landmark events (Loftus & Marburger, 1982) and reducing the amount of time that elapses between event and measurement, among other factors (Schwarz & Sudman, 1996).

Questionnaires

All aspects of the questionnaire (i.e., questions; response categories; question order; and for self-administered questionnaires, format and appearance) can influence both responses as well as the respondents' willingness to complete the survey.[5] Several fundamental problems with item design (e.g., questions and response categories) recur frequently. For example, consider the following question:

> Did the surgeon explain the risks and benefits of the surgery in a way you could understand?
> > 1 = YES
> > 2 = NO

The question is double-barreled; it asks about both risks and benefits in the same question. It would be hard to interpret the responses. Does a "yes" mean either or both? To fix this problem, we would ask one question about risks and another question about benefits.

When utilizing established scales, issues associated with question order, question content, response categories, and scaling have already been worked through; basically, what remains is the desired formatting of the instrument (such as a booklet for a mail survey, or writing a computer-assisted telephone interviewing [CATI] program for telephone administration). However, when questions are created from scratch, careful attention must be paid to question wording and the response alternatives (Rockwood, Sangsterd & Dillman, forthcoming).

Several issues are associated with item construction and ordering. The scope of a question can vary from the evaluation of discrete events (such as explaining the risks associated with surgery) to global evaluations (e.g., If you had to do it over again, would you come back to this institution for your surgery?). The nature of the requested evaluation can vary. For example, the dimensions might include frequency of occurrence (e.g., How often did nurses check on how you were doing?) or level of satisfaction (e.g., How satisfied were you with how often nurses checked on how you were doing?). Although these questions target the same event, they do so in different ways and can produce different responses. The location of questions in the instrument also can influence response (Schul & Schiff, 1993; Schuman & Presser, 1981).

The final challenge lies in interpreting responses to a question. For example, giving items a rating based on a level of satisfaction produces only a ranking. The actual importance of these items is unknown, so it is hard to interpret the meaning of the satisfaction rating. Although many satisfaction scales seem to use some form of weighted response metric, it is difficult to anchor the level of satisfaction in everyday life, especially in light of positive response bias. One way to approach this dilemma is by asking respondents to provide their own norms. For example, they could be asked to indicate the importance of various attributes of care and then subsequently asked to rate their availability. The importance serves as a basis for weighting the individual items, but other parameters could also be used.

ARE EXISTING SATISFACTION MEASURES AVAILABLE FOR RESEARCHERS?

Good measures of patient satisfaction are hard to find. Many extant questionnaires seem to be variants of a few basic works, many of which can be traced back to the early studies of Ware, Snyder, and Wright (1976). Few of these scales have been well tested to establish their psychometric properties or to define with which groups of patients they work best.

The two most utilized patient (consumer) satisfaction surveys, either in full or in part, are the Group Health Association of America (GHAA) Consumer Satisfaction Survey (Davies & Ware, 1991) and the Picker/Commonwealth survey (Gerteis et al., 1993; Picker Institute, 1992). A special effort is currently underway to develop satisfaction measures that can be used in the context of managed care.

GHAA Survey

The GHAA survey was developed primarily for employers that offer their employees one or more health benefit options and want to obtain valid and comparable health benefit options. The base GHAA instrument contains 60 questions, which are broken into the following sections in the survey instrument: satisfaction with health care services and providers, general satisfaction with care, satisfaction with health plan, health insurance and use of services, and personal characteristics. (An additional module assesses satisfaction with a specific visit.) From the instrument, 11 multi-item scales and 6 single-item scales have been developed. The content of each of the subscales is analyzed as follows:

- *Multi-item scales:* Access, finances, technical quality, communication, choice and continuity, interpersonal care, services covered, information, paperwork, costs of care, general satisfaction
- *Single-item scales:* Overall care, time spent, outcomes, overall quality, overall plan, plan satisfaction

Four separate evaluations were carried out to evaluate the psychometric properties of the subscales in the instrument. As expected, the responses were skewed positively, but the researchers concluded that the effect, while present, was not so marked as to be worrisome. (Davies & Ware, 1991). To assess *construct validity*, the hypothesized correlations between the individual items and all scales were examined. Most items in the survey demonstrated their highest correlations with the expected scale. The internal consistency of the multi-item scales was evaluated using Cronbach's alpha. The alphas for all the multi-item scales were in the acceptable range (.80 to .97).

In addition to face validity, the correlations between whether the person would recommend his or her health plan to others and whether he or she intended to switch health plans at the next available opportunity were examined. The predicted pattern, that lower ratings would predict a lower probability of recommendation and a higher probability of switching plans, was found.

The GHAA survey strengths include the breadth of topics addressed and its utilizability by hospitals, providers, employers, and insurers. It addresses the development and scoring of variables and recommends an analysis plan for survey data. It also utilizes an excellent–poor Likert-type response set, which Ware and Hays (1988) revealed as superior to strongly agree–strongly disagree metrics. The largest weakness is the lack of specific measures about outpatient services. However, the questions and outcomes measures from the five sections can be revised for an outpatient setting. Although it was designed to assess satisfaction with managed care, it has been adapted for other purposes, not always appropriately.

Picker/Commonwealth

The Picker/Commonwealth hospital satisfaction survey was developed as part of a larger initiative to emphasize patient-centered care. Obtaining information from patients' perspectives and relevant to patients' real concerns, expressed in terms that are meaningful to them, is central to this effort. Although much of the work has occurred within the institutional setting, the goal is an overall model for the delivery of health care at all levels. There are seven fundamental aspects to this model of patient care (Gerteis et al., 1993).

1. respect for patients' values, preferences, and expressed needs
2. coordination and integration of care (including clinical care, ancillary and support services, and front-line care)
3. information, communication, and education
4. physical comfort (including not just pain, but also a focus on institutional surroundings, such as hospital rooms, clinic examining rooms, etc.)
5. emotional support and acknowledgment of patients' fears/anxieties
6. involvement of family/friends in patients' care
7. transitions in care that ensure continuity

A series of 52 questions was developed to explore specific action taken by the hospital staff. Most of the response options were dichotomous, but follow-up questions were sometimes used to elicit more information about the problems reported. General headings include the following:

- communication
- financial information
- patients' needs and preferences
- emotional support
- physical comfort
- pain management
- education
- family participation
- discharge preparation/continuity of care

In the overall survey of 6,455 patients discharged from 62 hospitals, at least 10% of respondents reported problems in half the questions posed (Cleary et al., 1991). In a subsequent analysis that focused on only nonsurgical patients, about the same rate of problems was reported, although the problem classification differed somewhat. (Delbanco et al., 1995).

Patient Satisfaction Scale

The Patient Satisfaction Scale (PSS) was developed to assess patients' perception of their physicians' communication abilities, affective behavior, technical competence, and the patients' general satisfaction with their physicians (DiMatteo and Hays, 1980). Their survey was tested on 287 primarily low-income patients in a family practice clinic based in a county hospital in 1978.

The PSS is comprised of 27 questions, 25 of which were related to the four subscales. Two additional questions asked about the physician's inquiry about the patient's family and job status, although these were not found to correlate with the other subscales. All questions were scaled on a five-point Likert scale. Eight questions asked about various aspects of the physician's communication ability. For example, patients were asked to indicate their level of agreement with the following statements:

- This doctor always gives me suggestions on what I can do to stay healthy.
- This doctor doesn't give me a chance to say what is on my mind.

The other six questions also alternated positive and negative wording to minimize the degree of acquiescence response bias (DiMatteo and Hays, 1980).

Nine quesions focused on the physician's affective behavior. For example:

- This doctor usually does not try to make me feel better when I am upset or worried.
- This doctor always relieves me about my medical condition.

Three questions asked patients about their judgment of the physician's technical ability:

- I have some doubts about this doctor.
- This doctor always seems to know what he/she is doing.
- I have a great deal of confidence in this doctor.

Lastly, five questions focused on the patient's general satisfaction with his/her physician. For example:

- I don't think I would recommend this doctor to a friend.
- This doctor is the nicest person I have ever known.

Internal consistency and test–retest reliability were evaluated for the four subscales and found to be reasonably high. The general satisfaction scale had a Cronbach's alpha of .76, while the communication, affective behavior, and technical ability subscales had Cronbach alphas of .75, .79, and .60, respectively. The test–retest reliability was only done on 24 subjects and ranged from .11 for the technical ability subscale to .66 for the communication subscale (DiMatteo and

Hays, 1980, p. 22–24). The Cronbach's alpha for the 25-item scale was .92, and the test–retest reliability score for the 25-item scale was .63.

Subsequent patient satisfaction surveys have been used, in part, on this survey, although the patient sample and year of its development limit its wholesale adoption for other populations today.

WHAT CAN BE EXPECTED FROM FUTURE MEASURES?

With the growing focus on managed care, the Agency for Health Care Policy and Research (AHCPR) is currently funding the Consumer Assessments of Health Plans Study (CAHPS). At present, the CAHPS project is partially through Phase 1 (of 2 phases). This 5-year study's overall goal is to provide an integrated set of carefully tested and standardized survey questionnaires and accompanying report formats that can be used to collect and report meaningful and reliable information from health plan enrollees about their experiences. These questionnaires are being designed for use with all types of health insurance enrollees (Medicaid and Medicare beneficiaries as well as the privately insured) and across the full range of health care delivery systems, from fee-for-service to managed care plans. Besides a core set of items designed for use with all respondents, additional questions are targeted for use with certain subgroups, such as persons with chronic conditions or disabilities, Medicaid and Medicare beneficiaries, and children.

The CAHPS questionnaires will collect data on the following:

- access, communication, and interaction with the health care professional
- continuity and coordination of care
- preventive care
- administrative burden
- health plan's customer service
- enrollment
- personal contribution toward the premium
- utilization of health services
- health status
- respondent characteristics

This survey, along with others developed along the same lines, adds to the range of experiences that can be assessed by consumers (Allen & Rogers, 1996). The measurement of patient satisfaction has the potential to expand the sources of useful information that consumers use in choosing health plans, physicians, and hospitals.

CONCLUSION

Patient satisfaction is an essential component of the outcomes of care. It is easier to acknowledge its importance than to decide how best to capture its nuances. Recently, much attention has been devoted to seeking accurate ways to reflect patients' perceptions. As with all measures, there is a delicate balance between summary generalizations and aggregations of specific elements. It is easier to use the former than to try to create empirical rules for combining elements to calculate the latter. Because words mean different things to different people, it is often hard to find sufficient common ground to ensure that comparable constructs are being tapped.

These difficulties come at a time when the salience of patient satisfaction is rising. A study on how consumers select a health plan suggested that most consumers are more influenced by the opinions of their friends than by empirical data about the effectiveness of the plan's care (Kaiser Family Foundation & Agency for Health Care Policy and Research, 1996). Much more work is needed to develop user-friendly satisfaction measures that can accurately and meaningfully tap the relevant dimensions of this important but elusive concept.

REFERENCES

Allen, M.M. Jr., & Rogers W. H. (1996). Consumer surveys of health plan performance: A comparison of content and approach and a look to the future. *The Joint Commission Journal on Quality Improvement, 22*(12), 775–794.

Arahony L., & Strasser, S. (1993). Patient satisfaction: What we know about what we still need to explore. *Medical Care Review, 50*(1), 49–79.

Aquilino, W.S. (1994). Interview mode effects in surveys of drug and alcohol use: A field experiment. *Public Opinion Quarterly, 58,* 210–240.

Aseltine, R.H. Jr., Carlson, K.J., Fowler, F.J. Jr., & Barry, M.J. (1995). Comparing prospective and retrospective measures of treatment outcomes. *Medical Care, 33,* AS67–76.

Babbie, E. (1992). *The practice of social research.* (6th ed.). Belmont, CA: Wadsworth Publishing.

Baddeley, A. (1979). The limitations of human memory: Implications for the design of retrospective surveys. In L. Moss & H. Goldstein (Eds.), *The recall method in social surveys,* (pp. 13–30). London: University of London Institute of Education.

Bartlett, E.E., Grayson, M., Barker, R., Levine, D.M., Golder, A., & Libber, S. (1984). The effects of physician communication skills on patient satisfaction, recall, and adherence. *Journal of Chronic Disease, 37*(9/10), 755–764.

Bradburn, N.M. (1979). *Improving interview method and questionnaire design.* San Francisco: Jossey-Bass, Publishers.

Brewer, J., & Hunter, A. (1989). *Multimethod research: A synthesis of styles.* Newbury Park, CA: Sage Publications.

Campbell, D.T., & Overman, S.E. (Eds.). (1988). *Methodology and epistemology for social science: Selected papers.* Chicago: University of Chicago Press.

Carey, R.G., & Seibert, J.H. (1993). A patient survey system to measure quality improvement: Questionnaire reliability and validity. *Medical Care, 31*(9), 834–845.

Carr-Hill, R.A. (1992). The measurement of patient satisfaction. *Journal of Public Health Medicine, 14*(3), 236–249.

Churchill, J.J., & Suprenant, C. (1982). An investigation into the determinants of customer satisfaction. *Journal of Marketing Research, 19*, 491–504.

Cleary, P.D., Edgman-Levitan, S., Roberts, M.J., Moloney, T.W., McMullen, W., Walker, J.D., & Delbanco, T.L. (1991). Patients evaluate their hospital care: A national survey. *Health Affairs, 10*, 254–267.

Cleary, P.D., & McNeil, B.J. (1988). Patient satisfaction as an indicator of quality care. *Inquiry, 25*, 25–36.

Cook, T.D., & Campbell, D.T. (1979). *Quasi-experimentation: Design and analysis issues for field settings.* Chicago: Rand McNally.

Davies, A.R., & Ware, J.E. Jr. (1988). Involving consumers in quality assessment. *Health Affairs, 7*(1), 33–48.

Davies, A.R., & Ware, J.E. Jr. (1991). *GHAA's consumer satisfaction survey and user's manual.* Washington, DC: Group Health Association of America.

de Leeuw, E. (1992). *Data quality in mail, telephone, and face to face surveys.* Amsterdam: TT Publikaties.

Delbanco, T.L., Stokes, D.M., Cleary, P.D., Edgman-Levitan, S., Walker, J.D., Gerteis, M., & Daley, J. (1995). Medical patients' assessments of their care during hospitalization: Insights for internists. *Journal of General Internal Medicine, 10*(12), 679–685.

Dillman, D.A. (1978). *Mail and telephone surveys: The total design method.* New York: John Wiley & Sons.

Dillman, D.A., Sangster, R.L., Tarnai, J., Rockwood, T.H. (1996). Understanding differences in people's answers to telephone and mail surveys. In M.T. Braverman (Ed.), *Advances in survey research: New directions for program evaluation, 70*, 45–62. San Francisco: Jossey-Bass, Publishers.

DiMatteo, M.R., & Hays, R. (1980). The significance of patients' perceptions of physician conduct: A study of patient satisfaction in a family practice center. *Journal of Community Health, 6*(1), 18–34.

Doering, E.R. (1983). Factors influencing inpatient satisfaction with care. *Quality Review Bulletin, 9*(10), 291–299.

Donabedian, A. (1966). Evaluating the quality of medical care. *Milbank Memorial Fund Quarterly, XLIV*(3), 166–206.

Gerteis, M., Edgman-Levitan, S., Daley, J., et al. (1993). *Through the patient's eyes: Understanding and promoting patient-centered care.* San Francisco: Jossey-Bass, Publishers.

Groves, R.M. (1989). *Survey errors and survey costs.* New York: John Wiley & Sons.

Groves, R.M., Biemer, P.P., Lyberg, E., Massey, J.T., Nichols, W. L. II, Waksberg, J. (Eds.). (1988). *Telephone survey methodology.* New York: John Wiley & Sons.

Hall, J.A., Milburn, M.A., & Epstein, A.M. (1993). A causal model of health status and satisfaction with medical care. *Medical Care, 31*(1), 84–94.

Hansen, M.H., Hurwitz, W.N., & Madow, W.G. (1953). *Sample survey methods and theory* (vols. I and II). New York: John Wiley & Sons.

Housten, C.S., & Pasanen, W.E. (1972). Patients' perceptions of hospital care. *Hospitals, 46*(16), 70–74.

John, J. (1992). Patient satisfaction: The impact of past experience. *Journal of Health Care Marketing,* *12*(3), 56–64.

Kaiser Family Foundation & Agency for Health Care Policy and Research. (1996). *Americans as* *health care consumers: The role of quality information: Report of a survey.* Menlo Park, CA: Kaiser Family Foundation.

Kane, R.L., Maciejewski, M., & Finch, M. (in press). The relationship of patient satisfaction with care and clinical outcomes. *Medical Care.*

Kennedy, M. (1996). Designing surveys for maximal satisfaction: An interview with Allyson Ross Davies. *The Joint Commission Journal on Quality Improvement, 22*(5), 369–373.

Kish, L. (1965). *Survey sampling.* New York: John Wiley & Sons.

Ley, P., Kinsey, J., & Atherton, S.T. (1976). Increasing patients' satisfaction with communication. *British Journal of Social and Clinical Psychology, 15*(4), 403–413.

Locander, W., Sudman, S., & Bradburn, N. (1976). An investigation of interview method, threat, and response distortion. *Journal of the American Statistical Association, 71*, 269–275.

Lochman, J.E. (1983). Factors related to patients' satisfaction with their medical care. *Journal of* *Community Health, 9*(2), 91–108.

Locker, D., & Dunt, D. (1978). Theoretical and methodological issues in sociological studies of consumer satisfaction with medical care. *Social Science and Medicine, 12*, 283–292.

Loftus, E.F., Klinger, M.R., Smith, K.D., & Fiedler, J. (1990). A tale of two questions: Benefits of asking more than one question. *Public Opinion Quarterly, 54*, 330–345.

Loftus, E.F., & Marburger, W. (1982). Since the eruption of Mt. St. Helens, has anyone beaten you up? Improving the accuracy of retrospective reports with landmark events. *Memory and Cognition, 11*, 114–120.

Marquis, M.S., Davies, A.R., & Ware, J.E. (1983). Patient satisfaction and change in medical care provider: A longitudinal study. *Medical Care, 21*(8), 821–829.

Pascoe, G.C. (1983). Patient satisfaction in primary health care: A literature review and analysis. *Evaluation and Program Planning, 6*, 185–210.

Picker Institute (1992).

Press, I., Ganey, R., & Malone, M.P. (1990). Satisfied patients can spell financial well-being. *Healthcare Financial Management, 45*(2), 34–36, 38, 42.

Rockwood, T.H., Sangster, R.L., Dillman, D.A. (forthcoming). The effect of response categories on questionnaire answers: Context and mode effects. *Sociological Methods and Research.*

Ross, C.K., Frommelt, G., Hazelwood, L., & Chang, R.W. (1987). The role of expectations in patient satisfaction with medical care. *Journal of Health Care Marketing, 7*, 16–26.

Ross, C.K., Steward, C.A., & Sinacore, J.M. (1995). A comparative study of seven measures of patient satisfaction. *Medical Care, 33*(4), 392–406.

Salant, P., & Dillman, D.A. (1994). *How to conduct your own survey.* New York: John Wiley & Sons.

Schul, Y., & Schiff, M. (1993). Measuring satisfaction with organizations: Predictions from information accessibility. *Public Opinion Quarterly, 57*, 536–551.

Schuman, H., & Presser, S. (1981). *Questions and answers in attitude surveys: Experiments on* *question form, wording, and context.* San Diego, CA: Academic Press.

Schwarz, N., & Sudman, S. (Eds.). (1996). *Answering questions: Methodology for determining* *cognitive and communicative processes in survey research.* San Francisco: Jossey-Bass, Publishers.

Shortell, S.M., Richardson, W.C., LoGerfo, L.P., Diehr, P., Weaver, B., & Green, K.E. (1977). The relationship among dimensions of health services in two provider systems: A causal model approach. *Journal of Health and Social Behavior, 18,* 139–159.

Singer, E., Von Thurn, D.R., & Miller, E.R. (1995). Confidentiality assurances and response. *Public Opinion Quarterly, 59,* 66–77.

Strasser, S., Arahony, L., & Greenberger, D. (1993). The patient satisfaction process: Moving toward a comprehensive model. *Medical Care Review, 50*(2), 219–248.

Sudman, S. & Bradburn, N.M. (1974). *Response effects in surveys.* Chicago: ALDINE Publishing Co.

Sudman, S., Bradburn, N.M., & Schwarz, N. (1996). *Thinking about answers: The application of cognitive processes to survey methodology.* San Francisco: Jossey-Bass, Publishers.

Tanur, J.M. (Ed.). (1992). *Questions about questions: Inquiries into the cognitive bases of surveys.* New York: Russell Sage Foundation.

Tse, D.K., Franco, M.N., & Wilton, P.C. (1990). Consumer satisfaction as a process. *Psychology and Marketing, 7*(3) 177–193.

University Hospital Consortium. (1995). *1995 Inpatient satisfaction survey.* University Hospital Consortium Satisfaction and Improvement Program.

Ware, J.E. Jr., Davies-Avery, A., & Stewart, A.L. (1978). The measurement and meaning of patient satisfaction. *Health and Medical Care Review, 1,* 1–15.

Ware J.E. Jr., & Hays, R.D. (1988). Methods for measuring patient satisfaction with specific medical encounters. *Medical Care, 26*(4), 393–402.

Ware, J.E. Jr., Snyder, M.R., Wright, R., & Davies, A.R. (1983). Defining and measuring patient satisfaction with medical care. *Evaluation and Program Planning, 6,* 247–263.

Ware, J.E. Jr., Snyder, M.R., & Wright, R. (1976). *Development and validation of scales to measure patient satisfaction with health care services: Volume I of a final report. Part A. Review of literature, overview of methods and results regarding construction of scales.* Springfield, VA: National Technical Information Service.

Webb, E.J., Campbell, D.T., Schwartz, R.D., Sechrest, L., & Grove, J.B. (1981). *Nonreactive measures in the social sciences.* Boston: Houghton Mifflin.

Wersinger, R.P., & Sorensen, A.A. (1982). Demographic characteristics and prior utilization experience of HMO disenrollees compared with total membership. *Medical Care, 20*(12), 1,188–1,196.

Wolter, K. (1985). *Introduction to variance estimation.* New York: Springer-Verlag.

NOTES

1. A detailed exploration of the strengths and weaknesses of each particular method is outside the scope of this book. Readers interested in the issues surrounding the relative merits of each method should consult basic research texts (e.g., Babbie, 1992; Campbell & Overman, 1988; Cook & Campbell, 1979; Webb et al., 1981) or works such as Brewer & Hunter (1989), which focus on the integration of multiple research methods.
2. Sampling frames are usually derived from institutional records (e.g., discharges, clinic visits) and are thus usually current and identify the entire population. Using such records will also reduce error due to noncoverage (Groves, 1989).
3. In some instances, this might be modified to exclude respondents who have died, but, as noted by Groves (1989), any adjustments to this value should be carefully scrutinized.
4. Nonresponse error is based on the assumption that those who responded to the survey differ fundamentally from those who did not. Although the actual error due to nonresponse is usually unknown, special research studies have shown that it can be significant (Groves, 1989).
5. For more information on questionnaire design, see the following: Bradburn, (1979); Dillman, (1978); Schwarz & Sudman, (1996); Tanur (1992).

Part II

Treatment

Isolating the effects of treatment lies at the heart of outcomes research. It is all the more surprising, then, that so little work has been done to develop a taxonomy of treatment. Although in some cases, treatment may be viewed as a black box, looking inside that box to relate the outcomes to specific aspects of care becomes an ever-greater need. The most familiar model for treatment is the use of medications. Concepts like dose-response are common in that context, but they are just beginning to be used in a broader context.

The most obvious components of treatment are dose, duration, and frequency—but other aspects may be important as well. For some types of care, who delivers it may matter. The setting in which the care is rendered also can play an important role.

A generic approach to classifying treatment is needed. This taxonomy can serve as the basis for standardized data collection to ensure that relevant aspects of treatment are addressed.

Although treatment is the independent variable of greatest interest, its effects are not always direct. It is not enough to isolate the effects of other variables; it also may be necessary to consider the possibility that the effects of treatment are mitigated by some of these variables. Such an approach will require more complex models that examine the potential interactions of treatment and other risk factors.

5

Treatment

Paul Hebert

CHAPTER OUTLINE

- What Falls under the Term *Treatment*?
- What Do Outcomes Researchers Compare in Treatment?
- How Do Outcomes Researchers Measure the Effect of Treatment?
- Interpreting the Treatment Effect: What Are the Pitfalls?

Consider two outcomes studies. The first is a typical randomized controlled trial of the effectiveness of a new antihypertensive medication. Investigators in this study collect baseline data on clinical and demographic factors relevant to hypertension and then randomize patients into a control group that receives a traditional therapy of diuretics and a treatment group that receives the new antihypertensive agent. Before the treatment is administered, the patients in the two groups appear to be identical across all known risk factors. At the end of several months, investigators obtain outcomes measures from the patients. The differences in outcomes measures between the two groups represent the difference in the effectiveness of the new medication.

The second outcomes study compares the outcomes of hypertensive individuals treated in a health maintenance organization (HMO) versus a traditional fee-for-service (FFS) setting. Investigators draw historical demographic and clinical information from providers under the two financial settings and calculate measures of initial disease severity, comorbidity, and relevant outcome measures. They then use statistical techniques to compare the outcomes of care provided to patients in these two groups. The analyses employed here must first account for the potential differences (both observed and unobserved) between the two groups of patients associated with their decision to enroll in one or another type of care system.

Both of these studies are examples of outcomes research, and, if properly done, each can provide valuable information to improve the lives of hypertensive individuals. However, they differ dramatically in their use of key concepts, such as the treatment, the treatment effect, and the basis of comparison. In the first study, the treatment is a medication; in the second, the basis of comparison appears to be a financial arrangement. This chapter provides a framework to reconcile these seemingly different forms of outcomes research. A taxonomy of treatment is lacking in the health services research literature. A systematic investigation of the structure of treatment is a crucial step toward an appreciation of the many different factors that play a role in producing observed differences in outcomes between two groups. Recognizing all of these factors and the potential confounding role they play will become increasingly important as more non-experimental and quasiexperimental research is conducted.

WHAT FALLS UNDER THE TERM *TREATMENT?*

A broad working definition for *treatment* is a direct change in the health environment of an individual for the purpose of improving the individual's health status. The *health environment* includes those physical and social factors that have direct and presumed causal impact on an individual's health status. Treatment, as defined here, has two basic components: (1) what was done (process) and (2) how well it was done (skill). When a treatment is administered to a patient, these two factors of the treatment interact with initial health status (i.e., prior to treatment) of the individual and contribute to a change in health status. These relationships are depicted in Figure 5–1.

The basic model depicted in Figure 5–1 is used throughout the chapter, with items added to it as complexity to the notion of treatment is added. Solid circles in the figure represent measured constructs, such as initial health status and terminal health status. Solid lines represent causal relationships among the constructs. For example, Figure 5–1 shows a causal relationship between the initial health status of individuals and their outcome health status. Treatment is depicted as intervening in the relationship between initial and terminal health status measures. The effect of the treatment will differ depending on the baseline characteristics of the patients. The effect of a drug, for example, may differ greatly between young and old patients.

This conceptualization of the treatment intervening with the initial health of the patient is certainly not novel or controversial. It simply suggests that patients of

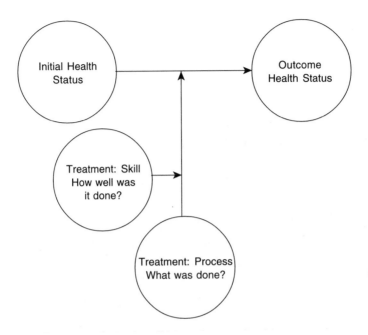

Figure 5–1 The Treatment and the Treatment Effect

various health states respond differently to the same treatment. Young patients respond differently from frail, older adults, and severely ill patients respond differently from mildly ill patients. Curiously, investigators do not generally use this framework in assessing the results of outcomes research. In general, researchers look first and foremost for a single, main effect of treatment. By comparing means of outcomes variables between the treatment and control group, or by examining a solitary coefficient on a treatment variable in a multiple regression, researchers attempt to discover the *treatment effect*—the main effect of treatment—and put restrictions on the statistical models that ensure the treatment effect does not vary with measures of initial health conditions in the model. Only after they discover a main effect do the investigators turn their attention to how the treatment effect differs across patient subgroups—that is, across patients of different health status. Investigators have adopted this practice, despite the fact that their original conceptualization of the problem suggests that the effect of treatment *should* differ importantly by patient health status. In fact, this hypothesized difference was one of the motivations for collecting patient baseline conditions in the first place. This perplexing lack of symmetry between the conceptual model of the experiment and the statistical techniques used to test its hypotheses is discussed in more detail in the later sections of this chapter.

The two dimensions of treatment are also depicted in Figure 5–1. Treatment is depicted as consisting of what was done and how well it was done. How well a treatment is administered modifies the effect of the treatment on health status. In quality of care terminology, what was done is often called *process* and is judged on the basis of its appropriateness for the situation. How well the treatment is delivered reflects the *skill of the practitioner* or the *quality of the equipment* used. For example, coronary artery bypass grafts (what was done) may have a positive impact on an individual with ischemic heart disease but only if the graft is sutured correctly (how well it was done).

Treatment: What Was Done?

The treatment of a disease or condition rarely consists of a single, isolated intervention on the part of the health care provider. It is better viewed as a continuum of interventions that, taken as a whole, define the treatment regimen. As depicted in Figure 5–2, the components of the regimen can be organized into three main categories: (1) medications, (2) procedures (including the use of medical devices), and (3) counseling or education.

These three categories are the basic building blocks of any treatment; they address what can be done to a patient in order to improve his or her health status. Assessing the outcomes of a treatment or a treatment group means examining how the care of a patient differs in quantity or quality across these three categories. Returning to the example of two outcomes studies cited at the beginning of the chapter, the financial arrangement (FFS versus HMO) that separated the treatment and control groups in the second outcome study is clearly not a treatment itself. Rather, the label *HMO* refers implicitly to the quality and type of medications, procedures, and counseling that characterize the regimen of care at the HMO. Using the financial condition as a basis of comparison implies that treatment regimens between HMOs and FFS arrangements differ in some ways that have implication for the health of hypertensive patients, even though the individual components that comprise the different treatment regimens are not necessarily observed.

Medications

Medications include not only prescription and nonprescription drugs, but everything that a patient physically takes into his or her system that has some causal, nontrivial relationship to health status. The type of anesthesia used during surgery, for example, could be considered medication. An outcomes study could compare the outcomes of patients who were given different anesthetics during

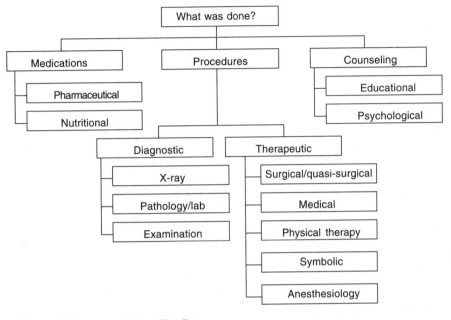

Figure 5–2 Treatment: What Was Done

surgery. The nutritional intake of patients could also be considered a type of medication.

An important aspect of medications as treatment is not only what medication was given but how much: the dosage. There are several ways to define the dosage.

- fixed dosage
- fixed dose per unit body mass or body surface area
- dose to tolerance
- dose titration until target outcome is achieved or a preset limit is reached

The dosage used is largely determined by the goals of the investigation (i.e., the basic research question) and the nature of the medication in question.

Procedures

Within the diverse category of *procedures*, it is important to distinguish between therapeutic and diagnostic procedures. Procedures that are purely diagnostic in nature do not seem to fit the definition of a treatment that was offered above. Diagnostic actions are treatments only to the degree that their performance changes the diagnosis and, hence, influences the treatment. For example, at first glance, a hemoglobin A_{1C} test does not seem likely to affect the health outcome of a diabetic patient (aside from the possible untoward consequences of drawing the blood sample). This procedure can, however, influence the health environment indirectly if it leads to a change in counseling, medication, or other procedure or if it has some symbolic psychological effect on patients' perceptions of their health. Using this or any other diagnostic procedure as the treatment in an outcome study could lead to ill-formed conclusions, such as hemoglobin A_{1C} tests cause diabetic shock, or mammograms cause breast cancer. Diagnostic procedures are better seen as a component of the skill of the provider—in particular, the intellectual skill of the provider—as discussed below.

Therapeutic procedures, in contrast, do have a direct effect on the health environment of the patient. A good starting point for a taxonomy of therapeutic procedures is the *Physicians' Current Procedural Terminology* (CPT) code (American Medical Association, 1994). The CPT is a listing of codes for medical procedures and services provided by physicians. It is developed and maintained by the American Medical Association in order to provide a uniform language that describes the medical, surgical, and diagnostic services a patient can receive from a physician. CPT codes are organized into six broad categories:

1. surgery
2. medicine
3. anesthesia
4. evaluation and management services
5. radiology
6. pathology and laboratory

The surgery category contains general surgical as well as "quasi-surgical" procedures organized by major organ system. Quasi-surgical procedures, such as percutaneous transluminal coronary angioplasty (PTCA), are used in lieu of traditional surgical procedures.

The medicine category contains several groups of procedures, some of which are diagnostic and some of which fall under the category of counseling. Medical treatments include dialysis, ophthalmological procedures, dermatological procedures, and rehabilitation procedures. Psychiatric services, which are listed in the CPT under medical procedures, might better be listed under the category of consultation/education. The anesthesia category includes services involved in the administration of anesthesia to patients.

The last three categories listed are not entirely procedures in the sense the term is used here. The evaluation and management services category, for example, includes primarily diagnostic consultative services provided by physicians. Many of these codes refer to face-to-face meetings between patient and physician that involve an examination and some medical decision making on the part of the physician but no treatment per se. Radiology and pathology services are similarly largely diagnostic in nature and are generally not considered types of treatment of their own.

On the other hand, comforting words from a provider, or a laying on of hands, may be an important form of treatment that affects a patient's recovery from an illness. In fact, not too long ago, this "art of healing" was considered the essential treatment a physician could provide. These "treatments" are labeled *symbolic* in Figure 5–2 and can also be provided with varying degrees of skill. Placebos should also be included in this category of symbolic procedures.[1]

Differences in both the type and quality of medical devices, such items as heart valves, pacemakers, surgical pins, braces, prosthetic limbs, and other durable items that replace or augment body functions, can affect the outcomes of care. Mechanical heart valves of various manufacturers and designs, for example, can display differing properties of thrombogenicity (the tendency to produce blood clots) and structural integrity, which can have an impact on health outcomes.

Counseling/Education

Counseling of patients refers to conveying to the patient information that is intended to change his or her health environment or behaviors. This category includes both psychiatric counseling as well as simple educational counseling, such as counseling a hypertensive individual on appropriate dietary changes.

Education can also be provided to health care providers in an attempt to change the treatments they provide to their patients. This education can take several forms. Direct education, such as continuing medical education or medical conferences, gives physicians and other providers information that can lead to a change in the type or quality of treatment they provide. Medical guidelines, practice parameters, and audit/feedback studies also represent educational treatments in the sense that they may have an impact on patient care.

A final form of provider education is cueing, in which physicians or other providers are given a cognitive cue designed to remind the physician to perform a desired procedure. For example, lower limb amputations among Native American diabetics were found to decrease when nurses serving the Native American community were instructed to have the patients remove their socks and shoes before seeing the doctor. The bare feet were a cue to the physicians to perform a foot exam. The treatment in this case is the education of the nurses. The effect on the health environment of the patients is any procedures, medications, or counseling provided by the physician as a result of the foot exam.

Other Treatments

More esoteric studies have included treatments that do not fit nicely into these three categories and perhaps deserve a category of their own. For example, studies on depression have used exposure to sunlight as the treatment of interest (Schwartz et al., 1996). Other studies have investigated third-party prayer as a form of treatment (Byrd, 1988; Marwick, 1995).

Treatment Regimens

Combinations of these basic building blocks represent *treatment regimens*. Outcomes research is often concerned with comparing the outcomes from one treatment regimen (i.e., combination of procedures, medication, and counseling) with those of another. Treatment from this perspective is sometimes viewed as a "black box" that contains all of the things that are associated with the overall treatment of interest. In the example provided at the beginning of the chapter, the treatment in the HMO group refers to a black box of various treatments provided by the HMO. Similarly, a study that compares outcomes of patients suffering from angina who receive drug therapy versus coronary artery bypass grafting (CABG) implicitly identifies the treatment in the CABG group to include all those medications, procedures, and counseling sessions that are associated with a CABG. As discussed below, how many of these correlated treatments researchers choose to consider part of the "treatment" dictates to some extent the conclusions that can or should be drawn from the study.

Treatment: How Well Was It Done?

The second critical aspect of a treatment is how well it was done. As Figure 5–1 shows, how well a treatment is done modifies the effect of the treatment on the patient's health status. The skill used to administer a treatment can be an important factor. The outcomes of care between two providers can differ substantially, even if both are adhering to treatment protocols deemed appropriate by previous research. This difference in outcomes is a reflection of the difference in treatment skill. Treatment skill can be deduced by comparing the outcomes among providers who offer appropriate care in similar settings.

As Figure 5–3 shows, there are several ways of looking at the skill of the provider. The first is *mechanical skill*. A researcher may be interested in whether a surgeon showed the manual dexterity to carry out a surgical procedure as it was intended. While surgery requires more than mere mechanical skills, a highly skilled surgeon in this respect may have very few complications due to poorly tied sutures or other surgical mishaps. *Mechanical skill* also refers to the quality of the

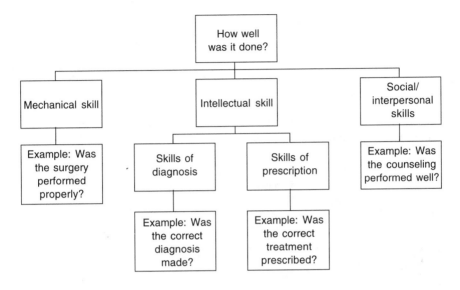

Figure 5–3 Treatment: How Well Was It Done?

medical device used as treatment. For example, high-quality heart valves with low profiles may decrease the incidence of thrombosis.

A second perspective on skill is *intellectual skill*. Here, the emphasis is on the provider's ability to reach the correct diagnosis and choose an appropriate course of action. A correct diagnosis is usually a prerequisite to choosing the right treatment. Timeliness may also play a role. In the example offered at the beginning of the chapter, differences in the outcomes in hypertensive individuals in different financial settings may be a function of the provider's ability to recognize the condition in the first place. How well the treatment was delivered is often a function of the elapsed time between the presentation of characteristic signs or symptoms and the initiation of treatment.

A third aspect is *interpersonal skill*, which includes the provider's ability to communicate with the patient. The communication may involve a straightforward transfer of information from the provider to the patient on how to monitor and maintain his or her health. Substantial skill is involved. Too often, what the provider thinks was said and what was heard by the patient are two very different things. The difference is a reflection of the skill of the provider or how well the educational treatment was provided.

The provider need not be a physician or even a health care worker. Pamphlets, videotapes, and interactive computer programs are all being used now to convey information to patients. The information content of the treatment (i.e., *what* is done) may be the same across all modes of communication, but the amount of information actually conveyed to and retained by the patient (*how well* it is done) may vary significantly.

Another form of interpersonal skill is the ability to console, reassure, or otherwise emotionally support the patient in an effort to bolster the patient's own healing mechanisms. The skill with which symbolic medical procedures are administered might be referred to as the *art of healing*. Until early this century, this aspect of treatment was considered at least on par with intellectual and mechanical skill. The president of Harvard Medical School in 1869 resisted a change in curriculum that would put greater emphasis on biological sciences on the grounds that the higher requirements might exclude natural geniuses in the art of healing (Starr, 1982).

WHAT DO OUTCOMES RESEARCHERS COMPARE IN TREATMENT?

Various factors can be used as the basis of comparing either what was done to a patient or how well it was done. Figure 5–4 depicts the relationship between the basis of comparison and other concepts in our simplified model of outcomes research.

The bases of comparison might be organized into the several categories shown in Exhibit 5–1. Although they are depicted as separate categories, they are not

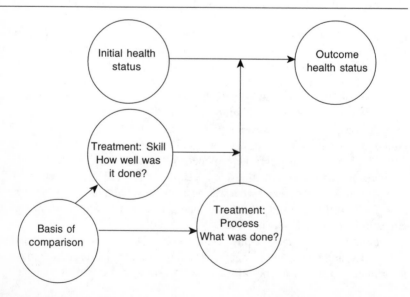

Figure 5–4 The Basis of Comparison

necessarily independent of one another. A difference in the outcomes of care across two hospitals, for example, is attributable not merely to the difference in physical setting but also to differences in the providers, the financial settings, the types and quality of treatments provided, and so forth.

Comparison of Different Treatment Regimens

A comparison of different treatment regimens is a comparison of what was done. As Table 5–1 shows, any treatment category (medication, procedure, or counseling) can be compared across this dimension. The cells in the matrix represent the various ways in which different treatments can be compared. Some of the cells of the table have been filled in with existing or proposed outcome studies as examples. Three dimensions of comparison are identified:

1. **Treatment A versus no treatment:** Do older adults who receive medication for isolated systolic hypertension have a lower incidence of cardiovascular disease than those receiving no treatment? Does counseling patients regarding treatment options improve patient satisfaction?
2. **Treatment A versus Treatment B:** Does CABG improve outcomes over angioplasty?
3. **Treatment A + B versus Treatment A alone:** Does an antihypertensive therapy of a diuretic plus a beta blocker reduce the incidence of cardiovascular disease relative to diuretic therapy alone?

Exhibit 5–1 Bases for Comparing Treatments

1. Comparison of different treatment regimens
   - Treatment A versus no treatment
   - Treatment A versus treatment B
   - Treatment A + B versus treatment A alone
2. Comparison of the intensity of treatment
3. Comparison of the duration of treatment
4. Comparison of the timing of treatment
5. Comparison of the setting of the treatment
   - Financial setting: e.g., HMO versus FFS
   - Physical setting: e.g., Hospital A versus Hospital B
   - Social/organizational setting: e.g., teaching hospitals versus community hospitals, hospice versus home care
   - Geographic setting: e.g., rural versus urban clinics
6. Comparison of the characteristics of the provider
   - Training
   - Experience
   - Personal characteristics

Table 5–1 Potential Studies of Various Treatment Regimens

	Basis of Comparison		
Treatment	Treatment A vs. no treatment	Treatment A vs. Treatment B (best current practice)	Treatment A + B vs. Treatment A alone
Medication	Systolic Hypertension in the Elderly Project (SHEP) trial. Investigated whether it is better to treat isolated systolic hypertension in older adults than to leave it untreated.		Should beta blockers be used in combination therapy with calcium channel blockers for patients with a history of myocardial infarction?
Procedure	Macular photo-coagulation study (MPS). Investigated the use of photo-coagulation vs. no treatment for eyes with choroidal neovascularization.	Are lumpectomies as effective as radical mastectomies in treating breast cancer?	
Counseling/ education of patient	Hypertension prevention trial. Addressed the effects of changes in health behaviors on controlling mild hypertension.	Is group counseling as effective as individual psychotherapy?	Does receiving physician counseling and watching videotape produce better patient compliance than receiving counseling alone?
Combinations			Is psychotherapy plus drug therapy more effective than drug therapy alone?

Investigators comparing treatment versus no treatment must take care to account for the placebo effect inherent in these experimental designs. The *placebo effect* refers to the phenomenon by which the patient's health status improves after being given a substance that has no metabolic significance. The patient reacts psychologically to the administration of the treatment, and these psychological changes affect the patient's physical well-being. If the treatment group is the only group to which a treatment is being administered, then changes in health status may reflect this placebo effect and not the effect of the treatment as envisioned by the researchers.

In many instances, investigators can control for the placebo effect by providing the no-treatment group with a placebo. In a drug outcome study, this would take the form of a benign pill that is similar in size and dosage to the medication in question but that has no significant metabolic effects. Developing a placebo for a procedure is more problematic, if not plainly unethical, as is the case for surgical procedures. However, researchers should attempt to minimize the placebo effect by having the control group engage in many of the same procedures associated with the treatment in question. If exercise with a physical therapist is the treatment in question, then researchers should have the control, nonexercise group members make the trip to the physical therapist even though they do not receive the treatment. Otherwise, the investigators could not determine whether any difference in outcomes between the two groups was not due simply to the fact that one group left the house and met with the therapist and the other did not.

Combinations of different classes of treatments can also be compared. For example, a study could address whether counseling on lifestyle changes plus drug therapy improves the outcomes of hypertensive individuals over drug therapies alone.

Since the critical issue in this basis of comparison is what was done, investigators should take steps to control how well the treatment was administered. For example, if the study compares one surgical procedure versus another, investigators should take steps to ensure the two procedures were performed by equally competent surgeons. A poorly executed CABG may have worse outcomes than a competently executed angioplasty, regardless of the merits of the two procedures. The effect of variations in the skill of the surgeon can be disentangled from the effects of the treatments by manipulating the experimental design or by accounting for these variations statistically. Solutions based on experimental design include randomizing surgeons to surgical procedures so that there is no systematic correlation between surgeon characteristics and type of procedure. Statistical solutions involve estimating a multiple regression, which includes dummy variables to indicate which physician performed the surgery. In this way, any special skills that a given surgeon brings to the experiment can be statistically disentangled from the effect of the surgery itself. Dummy variables that represent interactions between the surgeon and the surgical procedure he or she performed also may be necessary if some surgeons tend to be skilled in one surgical procedure but not the other.

Comparison of the Intensity of Treatment

Treatment intensity, that is, the amount of treatment per unit (i.e., per unit time, dosage, or encounter)—can have an impact on the effect of the treatment. Table 5–2 depicts various studies that compare treatments according to intensity,

Table 5–2 Potential Studies of Treatment Intensity

	Basis of Comparison		
Treatment	Intensity	Timing	Duration
Medication	Do higher dosages of diuretics reduce the risk of cardiovascular disease?	Is three times a day better than one?	Is ten days of treatment more effective than three?
Procedure	Does more strenuous rehabilitation improve recovery from surgery?	Does immediate post-operative rehabilita-tion improve recovery from knee surgery?	
Counseling/ education of patient/provider			Do longer counseling sessions improve the outcomes of psychotherapy?
Combinations	Diabetes Control and Complications Trial (DCCT) (Research Group, 1993) investigated the effect of more intensive treatment of diabetes.	Does early adjuvant treatment of cancer improve survival?	

timing, and duration. For example, studies of the effect of different dosages of medications, intensity of rehabilitation, or scope of counseling would fall under this basis of comparison.

Comparisons based on the duration of treatment could look at how long-term steroid use affects kidney function (medications), how more time spent in rehabilitation affects functioning after hip replacement (procedure), or how a greater amount of time spent educating a patient affects his or her health behaviors (counseling). In comparing across this dimension, both the type and the quality of treatment are of interest. For example, a brief counseling session may contain just as much information as a longer session, but it may not be conveyed as well.

Comparison of the Treatment Setting

The setting of the treatment—that is, where and under what conditions the treatment is given—can affect both the treatment regimen as well as the quality or skill of treatment. Studies that take the setting of treatment as the basis of comparison typically treat the treatment as a black box. That is, the investigators take as a given that treatment may differ qualitatively across settings, but they are not immediately interested in characterizing these differences. Rather, they concentrate on the implications of the differences (whatever they may be) for the health of patients in each setting.

Several aspects of treatment setting have been studied in terms of their impact on treatment and outcomes. The *financial setting of the treatment* refers to the method by which the providers of the treatment are paid for their services. Financial reimbursement schemes can have a substantial impact on the type of treatments provided and on the locus of care. The restrictions that HMOs may place on access to specialists have implications for the type of care provided to HMO enrollees. Similarly, changes in the reimbursements of hospitals over the last decade moved substantial amounts of care from inpatient to outpatient facilities.

The geographic and physical settings also clearly affect the type and quality of treatments offered to patients. For example, comparing surgical outcomes between rural and urban hospitals may reflect differences in care and available resources. Similarly, a comparison of outcomes between teaching and nonteaching hospitals tests the effect of the social and organizational setting on the outcomes of care.

Comparison across Providers of the Treatment

Figure 5–5 provides a classification of the various aspects of the provider of the treatment that can be used to compare treatment. *Orthodoxy* refers to the perspective of medicine under which the provider of treatment has trained. For example, chiropractors and neurologists both treat back ailments but have been trained under quite different philosophies. Consequently, the treatments they provide differ in type and perhaps quality. Another aspect of training orthodoxy is the treatment paradigm or practices of the institution where a provider trained. Certain institutions may emphasize preventive care, or cost-conscious medicine, or other treatment paradigms that are imbued in their graduates. Table 5–3 shows how the orthodoxy, as a basis of comparison, relates to the treatment regimen prescribed.

The *level of training* refers to the amount of time a provider spends in formal education (including clinical training). A board-certified specialist has more formal training than a general practice physician, and this training may affect the type and quality of treatment he or she provides. Table 5–4 speculates how training may affect the quality of a consultation between a patient and physicians with different levels of training.

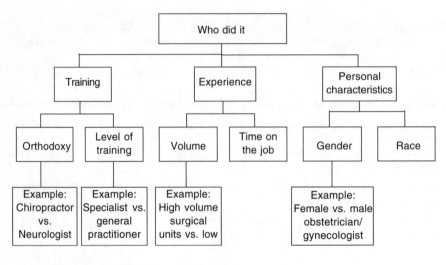

Figure 5–5 Aspects of the Treatment Provider

The effect of the provider's experience on treatment can be disentangled into the effect attributable to volume of treatment and the effect attributable to age—that is, accumulated practical knowledge and time since formal training. Volume can affect the intellectual and mechanical skill with which a treatment is performed. Low-volume surgical units are more likely to suffer from low quality than more actively used units (Shook et al., [1996]; Hannan et al., [1995]; Jollis et al., [1994]). A provider's age may have conflicting influences on treatment, since it may reflect either an accumulation of working knowledge or an unfamiliarity with the most recent findings.

Personal characteristics of the provider may also affect both the quality and type of treatment provided. For example, the gender of physicians has been associated with the frequency of Pap smears and mammography provided to female patients (Lurie et al., 1993). Patients who were treated by female physicians were more likely to receive these diagnostic procedures than were patients

Table 5–3 Differences in Treatment Associated with Provider Orthodoxy

	Orthodoxy of Provider	
Treatment	Chiropractor	Neurologist
Medication	Over-the-counter medications	Prescription medications
Procedure	Manipulations of the spine	Surgery
Counseling	High emphasis	Less emphasis

Table 5–4 Possible Differences in Treatment Quality Associated with the Provider's Training

	Training of Provider	
Quality/Skill of Treatment	*Specialist*	*General Practice*
Mechanical	High	Moderate/low
Intellectual	High	Moderate
Interpersonal	Moderate	High

treated by male physicians, although this difference ameliorated with the age of the physician. These results are difficult to interpret. They could reflect a reluctance on the part of either the patient or the physician to discuss sex-related issues with an individual of the opposite gender. On the other hand, the results may reflect a lack of vigilance on the part of male physicians to the needs of female patients. Alternatively, they may reflect the effects of a selection process whereby female patients who are concerned about prevention may seek out female physicians.

Figure 5–6 puts these various dimensions of treatment together. Across one axis is the type of treatment (medication, procedure, counseling, and combination); across the second axis is how well the treatment was done. The third displays the basis of comparison.

HOW DO OUTCOMES RESEARCHERS MEASURE THE EFFECT OF TREATMENT?

There are two basic approaches to measuring the treatment effect: experimentation and statistical analyses. Although these practices differ in method, the goal of each technique is the same: to create treatment groups in such a way that no unmeasured risk factors or important variables are disproportionately represented in any treatment group. If there is nothing different between the treatment groups except the treatment in question, then any difference in outcome measures between the groups can logically be attributed to the effect of the treatment.

Figures 5–7 through 5–10 show several ways that an unmeasured factor can enter into an outcomes study. An unmeasured factor is represented by a broken-line circle. A broken line with arrows pointing in both directions signifies an undetected, noncausal correlation between the factor and another element in the model. Broken arrows signify an undetected but causal correlation between the factors. Figure 5–8 depicts an unmeasured risk factor that is correlated with both patient characteristics and outcomes but not with the choice of treatment. (The goal of randomization to treatment groups is to create such a situation.) For

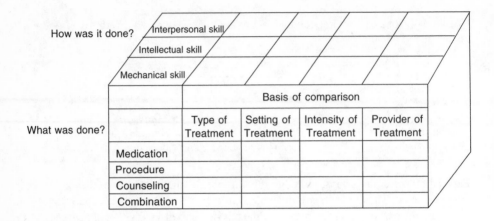

How was it done?

Interpersonal skill

Intellectual skill

Mechanical skill

What was done?

Basis of comparison				
	Type of Treatment	Setting of Treatment	Intensity of Treatment	Provider of Treatment
Medication				
Procedure				
Counseling				
Combination				

Figure 5–6 Treatment and the Bases of Comparison

example, both treatment groups may contain smokers, but smokers are not disproportionately represented in any treatment group. In this situation, the investigators may be able to discern the effect of the treatment in question.

Figure 5–9 depicts a more serious situation, in which the unmeasured factor is correlated with one of the treatments and the outcome but not with the underlying health characteristics of the patients in the treatment or control groups. For example, a patient enters a hospital for a given surgery and then is discharged to a rehabilitation facility. The quality of the surgery, the quality of the discharge planning, and the quality of the rehabilitation facility are all intrinsically linked. The investigator risks attribution bias by falsely attributing a difference in outcomes to one aspect of treatment (i.e., the surgery) when, in truth, the difference in outcome may not have been due to surgery but poor discharge planning or poor rehabilitation.

The situation is even more complex when the treatment is correlated with lifestyle changes on the part of the patients. Consider a study that compares nonsurgical and surgical treatment of ligament damage in the knee. After the treatment, the individuals may adopt significantly different lifestyles. Because individuals in the nonsurgery group have unrepaired knee ligaments, they may refrain from certain types of activities, whereas individuals who have had the ligament repaired may return to their previous activities. Even if individuals were identical before assignment to surgical and nonsurgical groups, after treatment they may no longer be equivalent. If individuals in the surgical group are found to have a higher incidence of readmission for knee injuries, it is not clear whether this would be due to a less effective treatment or to their more aggressive lifestyle following surgery.

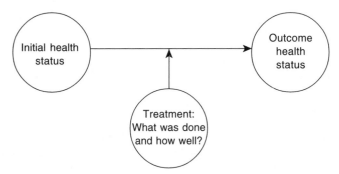

Figure 5–7 No Unmeasured Factors

There are two ways to lessen attribution bias in outcomes research. The first is to define accurately exactly what is and is not a part of the treatment and to measure all those factors correlated with treatment but not considered a component of the treatment effect. If the underlying research hypothesis suggests that correlates to treatment should not be reported as an effect of treatment, then these correlates should be measured and accounted for statistically. Multiple regression analysis may be able to disentangle the effects of the treatment from the effects of those factors that are correlated with treatment, as long as the two are not too highly correlated. That is, if every time treatment A is given, treatment B is also present and vice versa, then it is impossible to disentangle the effects due to A alone from the overall effects of A and B.

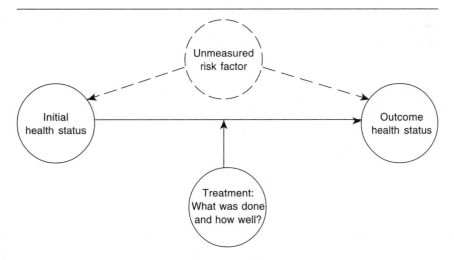

Figure 5–8 Unmeasured Factor Uncorrelated with Treatment

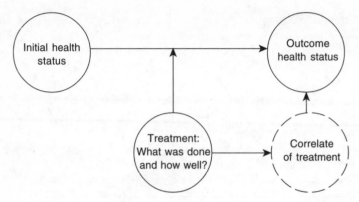

Figure 5–9 Unmeasured Factor Associated with Both Treatment and Outcome (Attribution Bias)

For example, two recent studies attempted to compare the outcomes of care provided by cardiologists versus general practitioners. The first study (Ayanian et al., 1994) examined the knowledge and practices of cardiologists versus generalists regarding drug therapy for acute myocardial infarction (AMI). The study found that cardiologists were more aware of drug advances than either general internists or family practitioners. The second study (Jollis et al., 1996) investigated the outcomes of AMI according to the specialty of the admitting physician and found that one-year mortality following AMI was lower for patients of cardiologists than for those of general practitioners. The basis of comparison in the second study is the training of the admitting physician, and the treatment is the

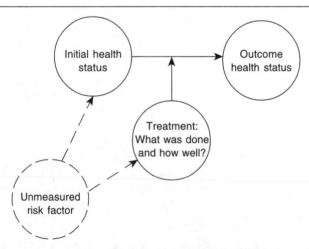

Figure 5–10 Unmeasured Risk Factor Associated with Initial Health Status and Treatment (Selection Bias)

combinations of medications, procedures, and counseling typical of cardiologists. The investigators found several variables that were correlated with the training of the admitting physician. For example, they found that cardiologists were more likely to practice in urban areas and to admit patients to facilities that had angiography available. They also found, like the first study, that cardiologists were more likely than other physicians to treat patients with certain medications that have been associated with improved post-AMI survival.

Which of these two factors, medications and angiography, should be "controlled for" in addressing the outcomes of cardiologists versus general practitioners? Both are correlated with the basis of comparison—that is, both are correlated with the specialty of the admitting physician—but are both part of the "treatment"? Should we control for availability of angiography by including it as an independent variable in a multivariate regression? The authors of the second study decided it was appropriate to control for the availability of angiography, but not for the use of medications. The purpose of the study was to investigate potential consequences of the recent trends by health care organizations to increase the use of primary care physicians and limit access to specialists. The authors of the study reasoned that the availability of angiography was not part of the treatment characteristic of a cardiologist, but perhaps an artifact of the tendency of cardiologists to practice in non-rural areas. Failure to control for the availability of angiography could result in a finding that cardiologists had superior outcomes, when in fact the superior outcomes were due to the availability of angiography. And, to the extent that differences in outcomes could be attributable to angiography, health care organizations should focus their attention on the availability of angiography, not on access to cardiologists.

The use of medications, on the other hand, was considered part of the treatment regimen of a cardiologist, and was not included as an independent variable in the analysis. Ayanian's study found that cardiologists have superior knowledge of the proper use of widely available cardiac drugs. This knowledge is a component of the skill of cardiologists. Controlling for the use of drugs would be like controlling for the skill of the provider, when the effects of differences in skill are precisely what you are interested in measuring. Thus, it would be inappropriate to control for the use of drugs in this study.

The second method of controlling attribution bias is to plan the timing of data collection to assess changes across the periods of interest. For example, if you are interested in the effect of alternative settings on rehabilitation from surgery (e.g., skilled nursing facility versus home care), then the initial health status, severity, and comorbidity measures should be taken at discharge from the hospital as opposed to on admission to the hospital.

Figure 5–10 shows the most damaging way in which an unmeasured factor can enter an outcomes study. In this scenario, some significant, unmeasured risk factor is correlated with the underlying health characteristics of the patient and the treatment in question. This clearly leads to biased estimates of the treatment effect. For example, if only the sickest patients receive a given treatment, then that treatment may appear to be less effective, or even harmful, relative to other treatments. In another example, physicians who are uncomfortable working with depressed persons may underdiagnose depression and be less skilled in providing the necessary care. This selection bias must be recognized and addressed either by experimental design or nonexperimental statistical techniques.

Experimental Techniques for Controlling Selection Bias

As discussed earlier, control and treatment groups should be constructed in such a way that the only difference between the two groups is the treatment itself. In this way, any observed changes in health status at the conclusion of the trial can be logically attributed to the intervention. When the investigator has control over the assignment of patients to treatment groups, the appropriate procedure is to assign individuals to the groups using some random process. The goal of randomization is to distribute patient characteristics equally across intervention and control groups. However, randomized assignment does not guarantee that the treatment and control groups are equivalent; it only provides some statistical assurance that the odds of nonequivalent control and intervention are small.

Stratifying

In studies with few patients, the probability that the control and intervention groups may differ according to some relevant variable can be significant. For example, if smoking is a known risk factor, then the investigators may not want to rely on chance alone to determine the distribution of smokers across treatment groups. Investigators can *stratify* on the factor to ensure that the same number of smokers end up in both groups. For more information on stratifying techniques, see Meinert (1986).

Single-Blind versus Double-Blind Assignment

Even when the process of assignment is based on some random process (e.g., a random-number generator, patient social security numbers, etc.), there is still a concern that knowing to what group a subject has been assigned may bias observations of the outcomes. As a result, researchers have adopted various ways of blinding the investigators to the assignment process. Random assignment can take two basic forms: *single-blind* and *double-blind assignment.* In single-blind assignment, the patient is randomized to a treatment or a control group, but the investigators take steps to keep the patients unaware of the group in which they were placed, lest the knowledge of which treatment they are receiving may induce patients to change their behavior in some way that jeopardizes the interpretation of the results of the trial. For example, the patient may become more attentive to the conditions that are known side effects of the treatment and report these conditions more frequently than had he or she not known the treatment being received.

In double-blind assignment, neither the patient nor the *investigators* (specifically, the individuals collecting and interpreting the outcomes and providing the treatment) are aware of whether the patient is in the intervention or the control group until the conclusion of the study. The investigators obtain consent from both the patient and any provider treating the patient before randomizing the patient into the control or intervention group. The investigators then take steps to conduct the trial without allowing the patient or the physician to discover the results of the randomization. The advantage of double-blind assignment is that it reduces the chance for bias introduced by the actions of either the patient or the care provider. If the physicians know that their patients are in the treatment group, and that the treatment is associated with certain side effects or outcomes, they might be more vigilant or attentive to those outcomes. Factors that may have otherwise gone unnoticed would be noticed and recorded by the physician, biasing the estimated incidence of that condition in the treatment group. In addition, the physician may unconsciously see one treatment as producing a better effect.

The disadvantage of double-blind assignment lies in the disinclination of both physicians and patients to participate in a trial without knowledge of which treatment the patient has received. This has led some to consider *prerandomized* designs (Ellenberg, 1984). In a prerandomization study, patients who have been deemed eligible are randomized into control and intervention groups *before* consent is sought from either the patient or the physician. If patients refuse to participate in the treatment regime to which they were randomized, they receive the alternative treatment (the control). Knowledge of which treatment group the patient will be in is expected to increase the number of patients willing to participate.

The goal of prerandomization is to increase the number of patients willing to participate to such an extent that it overcomes the dilution of statistical power due to potential selection bias. Specifically, patients who refuse the treatment may differ from the study population in some systematic way. The only way to combat this potential selection bias is to treat those patients as if they had actually received the treatment they were originally assigned. Analyzing the results of the trial based on the "intention to treat," rather than the actual treatment, has the effect of biasing the estimated treatment effect toward zero, making it more difficult to find a statistically significant treatment effect. However, this dilution of treatment effect can be partially compensated for by inflating the sample size (Zalen, 1977).

Natural Experiments

Natural experiments refer to situations where an intervention and a control group are created through some natural, systemic process, but that process is believed to be unrelated to the underlying characteristics of the patients. Since the process is unrelated to patient characteristics, the two groups are believed to be similar except for the intervention in question, and, thus, any difference in outcomes between the two groups is assumed to be attributable to the intervention. For example, a study of the outcomes of patients in coronary care unit versus non–coronary-care unit wards was conducted using data from a natural experiment (Chalmers et al., 1983). The investigators found patients who had been assigned to a coronary care unit but were not admitted because there was insufficient room in the coronary care unit. The process by which the patients got into the control or intervention group was based on the availability of a coronary care unit bed, which is unrelated to the health characteristics of the patient.

The advantage of natural experiments over traditional experiments is that, because they are historical accidents, they require no prior patient consent. This omission could increase the number of patients available for the study, especially when the treatment is a sensitive issue, such as access to a coronary care unit. The disadvantage is twofold. First, there is no real assurance—not even statistical assurance—that the process generates equivalent groups. A study of bias in treatment assignment in clinical trials of acute myocardial infarction found that at least one prognostic variable was maldistributed between the treatment and control groups in 58.1% of the nonrandomized trials studied (Chalmers et al., 1983). Second, natural experiments occur infrequently.

Nonexperimental Statistical Control of Selection Bias

In most instances, investigators do not have control over the assignment process and must rely on statistical techniques to create the treatment and control groups. There are two basic ways to do this: measurement of confounding factors and selectivity correction using instrumental variables.

The Creation of Equivalent Groups by Measuring Confounding Factors

Often in outcomes research, the comparison groups of interest were created neither by direct experimental control nor by a natural process that would suggest equivalent groups. For example, a historical comparison of surgical outcomes between patients of two surgical units cannot assume that patients of the two units were similar prior to surgery. In order to make meaningful comparisons of the outcomes of the two units, the investigator must measure and statistically account for differences in initial patient health status. Techniques for doing this have been discussed in previous chapters.

Having measured the relevant variables, investigators use multivariate regression analysis to disentangle the effect of the treatment on health outcomes from the contribution of these other factors that may affect the outcome. A number of good texts discuss the use of multivariate regression analysis in this context (Hirsch & Riegelman, 1996; Kennedy, 1993), and this extensive topic will not be covered here in any detail. Generally, however, convention holds that investigators estimate an equation of the form:

Outcome $_i$ =
$\beta_0 + \beta_1 \text{DEMOG}_i + \beta_2 \text{COMORBID}_i + \beta_3 \text{SEVERITY}_i + \beta_4 \text{TREATMENT}_i + e_i$
where

Demog = One or many variables representing Patient i's demographic characteristics, such as age, race, gender, and other fixed attributes that may be related to the outcome variable.

Comorbid = A measure of comorbid conditions for Patient i, as described in Chapter 7.

Severity = Measures of the severity of illness for Patient i, as discussed in Chapter 6. These variables can include severity indexes as well as other variables representing the baseline health status of individuals, including baseline values (i.e., pretreatment values) for the outcome variables.

Treatment = A variable that is equal to 1 if the patient received the treatment and 0 otherwise.

e_i = A random error.

Curiously, this conventional form of the outcomes equation is at odds with the conceptual model presented throughout this chapter. Specifically, this equation describes the treatment effect as a single effect, measured by the coefficient β_4, which applies equally to all patients, regardless of their initial health status. The model suggests that initial health status as measured by the comorbidity and severity variables does affect the outcome variable but that initial health status has no mitigating effect on the effect of treatment. That is, the amount of improvement in the outcome variable due to the treatment is the same, regardless of the initial health status of the patient. This is clearly at odds with the accepted clinical conceptualization of the effect of treatment, yet it is standard practice in outcomes research.

This convention is not limited to studies that employ techniques of multiple regression analysis. Traditional randomized controlled trials (RCTs)—the wellspring of scientific knowledge, from most clinicians' perspectives—also display this curious inconsistency. RCTs report the difference in the mean outcome between two groups as the treatment effect. This treatment effect is reported as if it applied to everyone in the treatment group. Data from a true RCT can be entered into a multiple regression and, assuming the assignment procedure affected a true randomization of all critical variables, the coefficient on the treatment variable would statistically equal the difference in the mean outcome between the two groups.

Of course, the cost of doing this simple comparison of means is low. A single, main treatment effect measure represents the average effect for all patients. Unless the treatment actually harms individuals with high initial health status and helps individuals with low initial health status (or vice versa), the interpretation of this main treatment effect is straightforward and unbiased. The only real cost lies in the fact that valuable information on the interaction of treatment with other variables is lost.

The equation below is conceptually isomorphic with the clinical model of the effect of treatment. Here, the treatment effect is measured as a main effect β_4 plus interactions with baseline measures believed to moderate the effect of treatment. The coefficients β_5 and β_6 measure how the effect of treatment changes with patient demographics (e.g., age) and changes in severity of illness, respectively:

$$\text{Outcome}_i = \beta_0 + \beta_1 \text{DEMOG}_i + \beta_2 \text{COMORBID}_i + \beta_3 \text{SEVERITY}_i + \beta_4 \text{TREATMENT}_i +$$
$$\beta_5 \text{TREATMENT}_i \times \text{DEMOG}_i + \beta_6 \text{TREATMENT}_i \times \text{SEVERITY}_i + e_i$$

where treatment is equal to zero if the patient is in the control group and 1 if the patient is in the treatment group. If the error from this regression (e_i) is uncorrelated with the treatment—that is, there is no unmeasured factor that is correlated with treatment and the outcome of treatment—then the coefficient on the treatment variable represents an unbiased estimate of the average effect of the treatment on the outcome.

The advantage of nonexperimental techniques such as these is that a wealth of historical patient data is available to the investigator, and there is no need for prior patient consent (although patient consent to be interviewed for outcomes information or even to review their medical records will still be needed). The clear disadvantage is that the investigator can control only for those variables that can be measured; there is no assurance that unobserved relevant variables are distributed equally across the intervention and control groups. Some common sense suggests the results of analyses such as this can be valid under these conditions:

• The risk factors for the condition under investigation are well known, and the investigators have measured them.

• There is little reason to believe that any unknown risk factor is correlated with one treatment.

Creating Equivalent Groups through Selectivity-Corrected Models

Selectivity-corrected models are a sophisticated form of multiple regression analysis that is appropriate when potential confounding variables are either unknown or difficult to measure. Selectivity models build on the basic model presented above by taking additional steps to ensure that unmeasured factors do not bias the estimates of the treatment effect. Given that this type of analysis has increasing importance to outcomes research, a heuristic explanation of selectivity correction techniques is provided. (For a more detailed discussion of selectivity correction, see Maddalla [1994]).

The most important element of selectivity-corrected models is the concept of an instrumental variable. An *instrumental variable* is some measurable event that gets individuals into a treatment group but has nothing to do with the health characteristics of the individuals. This is not dissimilar to the random-number generator that assigns individuals to treatment and control groups in an RCT. The results of the random-number generator determine whether an individual is assigned to the treatment group but have nothing whatsoever to do with the underlying characteristics of that individual. If an investigator can identify a naturally occurring variable or variables that fit these characteristics, then a selectivity-corrected model may produce unbiased estimates of the treatment effect.

For example, a study of the effect of more aggressive treatment of coronary artery disease (CAD) after myocardial infarction (MI) used the distance from the patient's home to the nearest hospital as the instrumental variable (McClellan, McNeil, & Newhouse, 1994). It was argued that, when a patient suffers an MI, he or she is taken immediately to the nearest facility, and the nearest facility[2] has nothing to do with the patient's underlying health conditions, but if the nearest facility engaged in aggressive treatment of CAD, then that patient was likely to receive more aggressive treatment.

The advantages and disadvantages of random and non-random construction of treatment groups are highlighted in Table 5–5.

INTERPRETING THE TREATMENT EFFECT: WHAT ARE THE PITFALLS?

Difficulties in interpreting the treatment effect can arise from problems at various stages in the study. Following Riegelman and Hirsh (1981), these stages are recruitment, assignment, assessment, analysis, and interpretation.

Table 5–5 Construction of Control and Intervention Groups: Advantages and Disadvantages

Assignment	Description	Advantages	Disadvantages
Random			
Single-blind	Patient randomly assigned to intervention or control group. Physician is informed.	No opportunity for bias in the interpretation of outcomes on the part of the patient.	Possibility of bias in the interpretation of outcomes on the part of the physician. Difficult to get consent of patient.
Double-blind	Neither physician nor patient know in which group the patient is.	Less opportunity for bias in the interpretation of outcomes on the part of the patient or physician.	Uncomfortable for physician. Difficult to get consent of patient.
Prerandom- ization	Investigator gets informed consent after he or she knows in which group the patient will be.	Physicians are more likely to approach patients to participate Patients are more likely to agree to participate.	Decreased statistical power. Opportunity for physician and patients to introduce bias.
Nonrandom			
Natural experiment	Patients are assigned to control and intervention group based on a natural process believed to be unrelated to the treatment of interest.	Many more observations available. Informed consent is easier to obtain post hoc. Fewer ethical problems.	Unobserved variables may cause bias in selection.
Equivalent groups	Control and treatment groups are formed by a nonrandom process, but confounding variables can be measured.	Many more observations available. Informed consent is easier to obtain post hoc. No ethical problems.	Unobserved variables may cause selection bias.

Recruitment Bias: How Did the Patients Get into the Study?

The first difficulty occurs at the point at which patients are recruited for the study. The risk here is that the patients are not representative of the general population of interest, and, thus, the results of the study may not be generalizable. Riegelman and Hirsch (1981) refer to this as *difficulties in extrapolation*—that is, drawing conclusions about the meaning of the study for individuals or situations not included in the study. Several factors may lead to recruitment bias:

- Subjects who agree to participate may be exceptional in their perceived need of experimental treatment.
- Subjects who agree to participate may be those who are least sensitive to the potential side effects of the treatment in question.
- Overly strict eligibility requirements may make the study population not representative of the general population.

Assignment Bias: How Did the Patients Get into the Intervention and Control Groups?

Assignment bias is introduced by a faulty procedure for creating treatment and control groups. As discussed above, this can often occur with nonrandom allocation procedures, but assignment bias can also be significant in randomized trials. A study on assignment bias in both randomized and nonrandomized studies showed that even in randomized trials, prognostic factors were not equally distributed across intervention and control groups, and the direction of the bias tended to favor the treatment group, that is, the bias would tend to increase the size of the treatment effect (Chalmers et al., 1983).

In double-blinded studies, 3.5% of the prognostic variables showed a statistically significant ($p < 0.05$) maldistribution between treatment and control, and this maldistribution favored the treatment group 56.1% of the time; that is, patients with favorable prognostic variables were assigned to the treatment group 56.1% of the time. These figures are reasonably consistent with what one would expect from a truly random assignment procedure. However, chance alone is unlikely to account for the maldistribution of prognostic variables in unblinded random assignment and nonrandom assignment. Approximately 7% of the variables in unblinded randomized trials were maldistributed, and 77.6% ($p < 0.001$) of the prognostic variables favored the treatment group. The figures for nonrandom trials were 34.4% and 81.4%. There is no way to test for randomization, but the results of the above study suggest that blinding the investigators to the treatment status at the time of assignment may improve the validity of the randomization procedure.

Compliance Bias: How Is It Known that the Treatment Group Received the Treatment?

Compliance may be a problem:

- Patients may lose interest in the study. This is especially problematic if patients discern that they are in the placebo group.
- Patients may be unwilling to tolerate the side effects of the treatment and may stop taking the treatment.
- Patients may be lost to follow-up: an extreme form of noncompliance in which the patient does not return for outcome assessments.

Compliance problems must first be ascertained before they can be improved. In trials of medications, the investigators can request that the patients bring in the bottle of medication they were provided in order to perform a pill count. Specialized medication dispensers can count the number of times medication has been dispensed. Direct testing of the presence of the medication in the body may sometimes be feasible, although expensive. (Some studies have added a harmless but detectable substance that permits compliance surveillance by urine samples.)

Regardless of the level of compliance, the outcomes data must be initially analyzed on an *intention to treat* basis. That is, even if there is reason to believe that a patient in the treatment group did not comply with the treatment protocol, his or her information must be recorded as an outcome for the treatment group. Treating noncompliance in this way yields a conservative estimate of the treatment effect.

Using intention to treat as a basis for analysis also accounts for complications of the treatment that limit compliance. If the side effects of the treatment are so severe or unpleasant that patients do not comply with treatment, fewer individuals in the treatment group will actually be receiving the treatment, and the difference between outcomes in the treatment and the control group will reflect this side–effect-induced noncompliance.

Analysis: How Were the End Points of the Study Ascertained?

As discussed above, patients or physicians who become unblinded to the treatment can change their behavior in ways that may bias the assessment of the end points (Meinert, 1986; White et al., 1992). In addition, inadequate concealment of treatment allocation among participating physicians is associated with larger treatment effects (Schultz, 1995). If the physicians know what treatment protocol an individual is assigned to, or if they know that a certain treatment effect or complication is believed to be associated with the treatment, they may be more vigilant in identifying problems or be more optimistic (or pessimistic) in assessing the outcomes. This could affect the reported incidence of the complication in the treatment group over the control, even though the true incidence may be similar across groups.

Interpretation: How Were the End Points of the Study Assessed?

The end points of treatment deserve thought. In some cases, the outcomes can be expressed as the results at follow-up. At other times, they are measured as a change score from some previous time point. Correct statistical techniques must be used to interpret the data collected in these various ways. This is a particular problem with nonexperimental studies where confounding factors such as initial disease severity and comorbidity may be correlated with both treatment and outcome.

CONCLUSION

This chapter's intention was to provide a framework for the analysis of the treatment effect across a wide range of outcome studies. Treatment has two dimensions: what was done and how well it was done. Outcomes studies assess the implications for patient health of changes in these two dimensions across some basis of comparison. Several bases of comparison were suggested, including what was done, who did it, and where it was done.

This chapter also discussed issues regarding the measurement of the treatment effect. In order to report an unbiased treatment effect, researchers must strive to create treatment and control groups that differ only by the treatment in question. Two ways of doing this were discussed: randomized controlled experiments and nonrandomized statistical analyses. Finally, difficulties in interpreting the validity of the measured treatment effect were discussed. Potential for bias can enter at any point in the study process. Investigators must be constantly vigilant to these various biases.

REFERENCES

American Medical Association. (1994). *Physicians' current procedural terminology (CPT)*. Chicago: Author.

Ayanian, J.Z., Hauptman, P.J., Guadagnoli, E., Antman, E.M., Pashos, C.L., & McNeil, B.J. (1994). Knowledge and practice of generalist and specialist physicians regarding drug therapy for acute myocardial infarction. *New England Journal of Medicine, 331*(17), 1,136–1,142.

Byrd, R.C. (1988). Positive therapeutic effects of intercessory prayer in a coronary care unit population. *Southern Medical Journal, 81*(7), 826–829.

Chalmers, T.G., Celano, P., Sacks, H.S., & Smith, H. Jr. (1983). Bias in treatment assignment in controlled clinical trials. *New England Journal of Medicine, 309*, 1,358–1,361.

Ellenberg, S.E. (1984). Randomization designs in comparative clinical trials. *New England Journal of Medicine, 310*(21), 1,404.

Hannan, E.L., Siu, A.L., Kumar, D., Kilburn, H., Jr., & Chassin, M.R. (1995). The decline in coronary artery bypass graft surgery mortality in New York state: The role of surgeon volume. *JAMA, 273*(3), 209–213.

Hirsch, R.P., & Riegelman, R.K. (1996). *Statistical operations: analysis of health research data.* Cambridge, MA: Blackwell Science.

Jollis, J.G., DeLong, E.R., Peterson, E.D., Muhlbaier, L.H., Fortin, D.F., Califf, R.M., & Mark, D.B. (1996). Outcome of acute myocardial infarction according to the specialty of the admitting physician. *New England Journal of Medicine, 335*(25), 1,880–1,887.

Jollis, J.G., Peterson, E.D., DeLong, E.R., Mark, D.B., Collins, S.R., Muhlbaier, L.H., & Pryor, D.B. (1994). The relation between the volume of coronary angioplasty procedures at hospitals treating Medicare beneficiaries and short-term mortality. *New England Journal of Medicine, 331*(24), 1,625–1,629.

Kennedy, P. (1993). *Guide to Econometrics.* Cambridge, MA: MIT Press.

Lurie, N., Slater, J., McGovern, P., Ekstrum, J., Quam, L., & Margolis, K. (1993). Preventive care for women. Does the sex of the physician matter? *New England Journal of Medicine, 329*, 478–482.

Maddalla, G.S. (1994). *Limited-dependent and qualitative variables in econometrics.* Cambridge, England: Cambridge University Press.

Marwick, C. (1995). Should physicians prescribe prayer for health? Spiritual aspects of well-being considered [news]. *JAMA, 273*(20), 1,561–1,562.

McClellan, M., McNeil, B.J., & Newhouse, J.P. (1994). Does more intensive treatment of acute myocardial infarction in the elderly reduce mortality? Analysis using instrumental variables. *JAMA, 272*(11), 859–866.

Meinert, C.L. (1986). *Clinical trials: Design, conduct, and analysis.* New York: Oxford University Press.

Riegelman, R.K., & Hirsch, R.P. (1981). *Studying a study and testing a test.* Boston: Little, Brown.

Schultz, K.F. (1995). Subverting randomization in controlled trials. *JAMA, 274*(18), 1,456–1,458.

Schwartz, P.J., Brown, C., Wehr, T.A., & Rosenthal, N.E. (1996). Winter seasonal affective disorder: A follow-up study of the first 59 patients of the National Institute of Mental Health seasonal studies program. *American Journal of Psychiatry, 153*(8), 1,028–1,036.

Shook, T.L., Sun, G.W., Burstein, S., Eisenhauer, A.C., & Matthews, R.V. (1996). Comparison of percutaneous transluminal coronary angioplasty outcome and hospital costs for low-volume and high-volume operators. *American Journal of Cardiology, 77*(5), 331–336.

Starr, P. (1982). *The social transformation of American medicine.* New York: Basic Books.

White, K., Kando, J., Park, T., et al. (1992). Side effects and the "blindability" of clinical drug trials. *American Journal of Psychiatry, 149*, 1,730–1,731.

Zalen, M. (1977). Statistical options in clinical trials. *Seminars in Oncology, 4*, 441–446.

NOTES

1. The use of placebos is complicated. The very act of treating a person, even ineffectually, may affect the outcomes of care. Placebo effects occur unconsciously and deliberately. In experimen-

tal studies, such as drug trials, placebos are deliberately used to control for the placebo effect. The degree of conviction a clinician brings to a patient can affect the extent of this effect. Presumably, a clinician in a drug trial, where the prescriber does not know whether the patient will receive a drug or not, will act with less conviction. In practice, clinicians' beliefs in the efficacy of their treatments can become a self-fulfilling prophecy with patients who are susceptible to placebo effects.

2. Specifically, the difference in the distance from the patient's home to the nearest facility minus the distance from the patient's home to the nearest "high intensive" facility.

Part III

Risk Adjustment

The goal of outcomes research is to determine the relationship between treatment and outcomes, but treatment does not work in isolation. Many other factors can influence the outcomes of care. A nonexperimental research design requires that special efforts be directed toward ensuring that any postulated relationship between a treatment and an outcome be assessed in the context of other factors that are associated with the treatment and control groups. Because clinicians and others are especially wary of the results of nonexperimental designs, where extraneous factors can be controlled, the burden of proof rests with the investigator. Adjusting for such potential extraneous factors–risk adjustment–is a crucial step. Risk adjustment is sometimes referred to as *case-mix adjustment.*

Risk factors may directly influence an outcome or may interact with aspects of treatment to produce their effect. Their influence must be assessed and proper adjustments made to avoid erroneous causal attributions. For example, older or sicker patients may respond differently to treatments. The credibility of a study may rest on testing for the effects of potential intervening risk factors. Thus, a policy of inclusion is often followed. It is better to test the effect of a potential risk factor and reject it than not to have considered it. The potential effects of risk factors can be tested only if they have been measured. A conceptual model of the factors believed to influence outcomes is critical, and careful planning is needed to ensure that analyzable data are collected on pertinent risk factors. Relying on routine clinical recording is unlikely to suffice.

Several classes of risk factors can be identified. The specific classification is arbitrary, and the lines separating one element from another often blur. Each of the three components of risk adjustment (severity, comorbidity, and demographic and psychosocial factors) is discussed in a separate chapter. *Severity of illness* addresses a set of descriptors that define the extent of a condition or the effects of that illness on the patient. It is effectively a classification for the patient's primary problem or the primary focus of the outcomes analysis. *Comorbidity* alludes to the potential effects of the presence of other clinical problems. Each of these comorbid problems may exist in various levels of severity.

The third cluster of risk factors includes *demographic variables* and *psychosocial factors*. While taking account of the effects of demographics seems almost instinctive because it is commonplace, careful thought about their potential role in causal pathways may uncover more subtle effects. Psychosocial factors may sometimes be outcomes in themselves, but they can also influence the effects of treatment on other outcomes. For example, depression may be an outcome of care, but depressed patients may not respond to care as well as those with a more positive attitude.

Understanding how various factors beyond treatment can affect outcomes is essential to such research. Social science theories can serve as a guide, but clinical insights are also important. Both should be employed in developing a conceptual model that describes the assumptions about what influences outcomes and how these factors might be related to each other. This model will drive both data collection and analysis.

6

Severity

Maureen Smith

CHAPTER OUTLINE

- Where Does Severity Fit in the Conceptual Framework?
- How Do Outcomes Researchers Choose a Severity Measure?
- What Specific Measures Are Available to Outcomes Researchers?

Researchers often wish to compare treatment outcomes for two or more groups of patients. Occasionally, researchers randomly allocate patients to each of the groups. More often, treatment groups are formed naturally through an unknown selection process. The problems generated by this selection process were brought to national attention when the Health Care Financing Administration announced that it would publish hospital mortality rates (Green et al., 1990). Many questions were raised about the quality of care provided by hospitals with high mortality rates. These published mortality rates also generated extensive controversy, particularly because the data did not control for the initial severity of illness of each hospital's patients (Iezzoni et al., 1992). *Initial severity of illness* can be defined as an estimate of the risk of an untoward outcome. If the rates were not adjusted for this initial risk, higher death rates in some hospitals might not necessarily represent poor quality of care. It would be unfair to identify and publicly penalize those hospitals whose results seemed poor because they were admitting the sickest patients.

In addition to being good politics, adjusting outcomes for the initial severity of illness is good science. There are several reasons to incorporate severity of illness measures into an analysis. These include adjusting for selection bias, improving the ability of the model to predict outcomes, and forming a basis for subgroup analyses.

All quasi- or nonexperimental designs must address the *potential for selection bias* when patients are not randomly allocated into treatment groups. Credible research will address this concern directly by measuring and adjusting for potentially confounding differences in initial severity. Although the researcher can never be sure that the relationship between the treatment and the outcome is not the result of differences in the initial severity of illness, risk adjustment based on initial levels of illness in each group can diminish this confounding effect.

Severity of illness is usually believed to be an important factor predicting outcome, whether or not there is any evidence of biased selection. In order to improve clinicians' confidence in the results, measures of severity are often included based on *a priori* beliefs that they will be helpful in explaining a high proportion of the variance in outcomes. These *a priori* beliefs alone are sufficient to justify the inclusion of these measures, despite evidence that severity measures do not in fact always explain a high proportion of the variance in outcomes when the data are analyzed. These severity measures may fail to explain much variance because the measures included in the study may not capture the important components of severity. Alternatively, factors other than severity of illness may be overwhelmingly responsible for explaining the outcome. Some of these other factors will have been measured, but most probably will not have been, and a high proportion of the variance in the outcome is likely to remain unexplained. Still, severity of illness measures should be included, given the overwhelming belief by most medical experts that they are theoretically important in predicting outcome and the propensity of those who may not agree with the study results to point to the exclusion of such measures.

The relationship between the intervention and the outcome may differ depending on the patient's initial severity of illness. For example, physical therapy may be useful for improving the functional status of stroke patients, but it may not be equally useful for all stroke patients. Patients who are completely comatose may benefit less from physical therapy than patients who are paralyzed but cognitively intact. This distinction illustrates the potential importance of *subgroup analysis*. Subgroups of patients with more or less severe disease may respond differently to an intervention. To avoid overanalysis of the data, subgroups selected for additional analyses should be identified prior to the beginning of the study and should be consistent with the conceptual model developed to explain outcomes.

In summary, important features of severity of illness measures include adjusting for selection bias, improving the ability of the model to predict outcomes, and forming a basis for subgroup analyses. The successful use of these measures depends on measuring all relevant characteristics of the initial illness in a reliable and valid manner and identifying appropriate statistical methods to test the hypotheses of interest. This chapter will focus on the first of these goals; appropriate statistical methods are described in a variety of other textbooks.

WHERE DOES SEVERITY FIT IN THE CONCEPTUAL FRAMEWORK?

An overarching conceptual model should be used to guide data collection and analysis for outcomes research. Placing severity of illness in this conceptual framework helps the researcher identify measures of severity most likely to be useful and methods for incorporating them into the analysis. In particular, linking severity measures to the domains of health identified in Chapter 2 reinforces the important message: a conceptual model of the outcome must drive outcomes research. Otherwise, important influences may be missed and the credibility of the research compromised. The lack of a conceptual model leaves the study vulnerable to post hoc reasoning. Outcomes research is more than explaining observed variation. It is best used to test beliefs based on clinical experience and theory.

Severity of Illness Measures and the Domains of Health

During data analysis, outcomes measures are adjusted for the potentially confounding effects of each group's initial severity of illness. The final outcome measures are often based on the concept of "health," which may include several domains. These domains were described in detail in Chapter 2, and include physical functioning, social functioning, emotional functioning, cognitive functioning, symptoms (or pain), and vitality. In contrast, traditional measures of severity are commonly based on the medical concept of physiological "illness." Most current conceptualizations of severity of illness include only one or two domains of health (Aronow, 1988; Pompei et al., 1991) This approach may have substantial limitations, particularly if omitted domains such as cognitive, emotional, or social functioning influence the final outcome measure.

Many traditional severity measures focus almost exclusively on the domain of physical functioning. For example, Pompei et al. (1991) suggested that physicians use several clinically defined concepts to relate a patient's initial level of illness at admission to the outcomes of hospitalization. These include the patient's overall condition, functional status, physiological severity of illness, burden of comorbid disease, and instability (i.e., ability to withstand an acute illness). Figure 6–1 shows the overlap between these clinically defined concepts and the domains of health described in Chapter 2. The majority of these clinically defined concepts of severity (e.g., physiological severity, comorbidity, and instability) are subcategories of the larger domain of physical functioning. Functional status tends to be

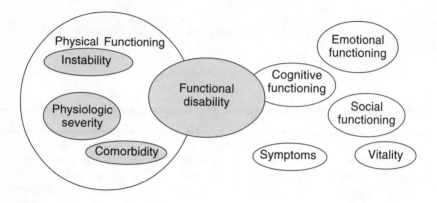

Figure 6–1 Clinically Defined Concepts of Severity and the Domains of Health

more inclusive; while it often focuses on physical functioning, other domains, such as cognition, may be implicitly measured as well.

By subcategorization, these clinically defined concepts convey more precise definitions for measures of the initial severity of illness. Nonetheless, the limitations of this approach are most apparent in its omissions. Major domains of health are excluded (e.g., emotional and social functioning). Many of these excluded domains have not traditionally been considered part of primary medical practice, and patients with these problems have been referred to other types of health professionals.

The conceptualization of initial severity of illness as domains related only to physical function may bias the conclusions of an outcomes research study. For example, clinical depression has been shown to worsen the outcomes of a number of conditions. For these conditions, ignoring the domain of emotional functioning may seriously hamper the ability to test the relationship between the proposed intervention and the eventual outcome. This potential bias may be addressed by developing a conceptual model of the outcome that explicitly considers the impact of each domain of health identified in Chapter 2. Iezzoni (1994) also has proposed a conceptualization of risk that explicitly combines the domains of health with the concepts of illness severity. In addition, she identified several other dimensions of risk, including the patient's age; sex; attitudes and preferences for outcomes; and cultural, ethnic, and socioeconomic attributes or behaviors. These demographic and psychosocial dimensions of risk are examined more closely in Chapter 8.

Which dimensions of risk are most important for adjusting outcomes? The answer varies depending on the outcome and disease of interest. Iezzoni (1994) suggests the "medical meaningfulness" test for assessing the validity of a risk adjustment approach. This test asks the following: Is the source of the risk (i.e., domain) linked to the outcome of interest? An evaluation of this potential linkage determines whether a particular risk adjustment strategy achieves validity and clinical credibility.

Components of Illness Severity

The components of illness severity that are most important for outcomes research are listed in Exhibit 6–1. The following conceptualization incorporates the domains of health, clinical concepts of severity (e.g. physiologic severity and comorbidity), and information about the patient's principal diagnosis.

General physiologic severity can be measured by variables that reflect basic physiologic functioning, such as heart rate, blood pressure, white blood cell count, and level of consciousness. These variables are scored identically for all patients, regardless of the principal diagnosis. Abnormal values of these variables reflect disorders of homeostasis and basic organ function. Traditionally, most severity of illness measures have focused on quantifying this component. These traditional measures are useful in classifying severity for acutely ill, hospitalized patients; they may be less useful in classifying severity in other settings, such as ambulatory care.

The *physiologic severity of the principal diagnosis* can be crucial to the eventual outcome. Most patients can be classified as more or less severe based on information specific to the principal diagnosis. For example, two patients with a diagnosis of breast cancer may vary dramatically in severity depending on whether the cancer is local or widely metastatic. For breast cancer patients, the most important classification of severity may involve the degree of metastasis. In contrast, patients with stroke may be considered more or less severe depending on the level of paralysis or loss of consciousness. In some cases, the components of severity will overlap. For example, loss of consciousness is a general measure of physiologic function, but it is also an extremely important determinant of severity for a patient with a principal diagnosis of stroke. For other cases, it may be difficult to identify a principal diagnosis, as in the case of older patients who have multiple coexisting conditions, such as diabetes, ischemic heart disease, and kidney disease. The presence of multiple diagnoses for a single patient necessitates additional identification and classification of these comorbid conditions.

Exhibit 6–1 Components of Illness Severity

- General physiological severity, irrespective of the principal diagnosis
- Physiological severity of the principal diagnosis
- Number and severity of comorbid conditions
- Baseline measures of the outcome domain
- Baseline measures of other relevant domains

The *number and severity of comorbid conditions* is a major component of the overall severity of illness. For example, in an otherwise healthy patient with pneumonia, the prognosis may be excellent. However, a primary diagnosis of pneumonia in a patient with acquired immunodeficiency syndrome (AIDS) or metastatic cancer may indicate an immediately life-threatening condition with an extremely poor prognosis. In addition, it may not be sufficient to identify the presence of a comorbid condition—the severity of the condition and its relationship to the primary diagnosis may need to be considered as well. A myocardial infarction in a patient with diabetes controlled completely by diet may have a relatively good prognosis; the opposite may be true in a diabetic patient with substantial end-organ damage, such as end-stage renal disease. In this case, the severity of the comorbid condition (diabetes) may dramatically influence a patient's life expectancy. The relationship of the comorbid condition to the primary diagnosis may also provide valuable information. Severe pneumonia in a patient with a primary diagnosis of low back pain has different implications from a severe pneumonia in a patient with a primary diagnosis of AIDS.

The outcome variable of interest may capture one or many domains of health. Incorporating a *baseline measure of the outcome variable* into a study improves a risk adjustment strategy for several reasons. First, it ensures that all domains included in that particular outcome measure are included in the measures of initial severity. Second, since the baseline measure is identical to the final outcome measure except for the timing of measurement, the variable is more likely to be measured consistently across the initial and final time periods. Unfortunately, while baseline measures are useful indicators of initial severity, it is not always possible or meaningful to collect them. For example, if the outcome of interest is death, the baseline measure is meaningless (since all patients are initially alive). However, if the outcome of interest is functional status (e.g., activities of daily living [ADLs]), a baseline measure can provide invaluable information regarding the patient's progress over time.

Baseline measures of other relevant domains of health (e.g., emotional, cognitive, or social functioning) can be equally important. Suppose the researcher wishes to study the relationship between occupational therapy (the intervention) and functional status at discharge from the hospital (the outcome). The relationship between the intervention and outcome may be substantially affected by the patient's initial cognitive status. For example, a patient with Alzheimer's disease may have a completely different response to occupational therapy when compared to someone who is cognitively intact. A baseline measure of cognitive functioning allows the researcher to incorporate this concern into the analysis.

It is important to note that, in practice, the five components of illness severity listed in Exhibit 6–1 are not mutually exclusive. For example, some severity of illness measures focus on general physiological severity but also include information about the patient's comorbid conditions. These five components are useful for purposes of discussion, but the real issue is whether the combination of severity measures chosen is appropriate and comprehensive enough for the task at hand. This chapter will concentrate on traditional measures of severity of illness, which usually incorporate elements of the first three components (general physiological severity, physiological severity of the principal diagnosis, and the number and severity of comorbid conditions). The measurement of outcome variables and other domains of health discussed in Chapters 2, 3, and 8 can also be used to characterize a patient's baseline status for purposes of risk adjustment.

Generic versus Diagnosis-Related Information

There has been much debate over whether severity is a generic or diagnosis-specific construct. There are three general types of measures (Iezzoni, 1994). First, *generic* measures rate the severity of a patient's condition using variables that are measured identically for every patient. The other two types of measures utilize diagnosis-related information. The second measure can be called *diagnosis specific*. This measure is developed only for patients with a certain diagnosis (e.g., patients with pneumonia). The third measure can be called *diagnosis considered*. It considers diagnoses by calculating severity ratings for each of a patient's diagnoses and combining all of the ratings into an overall score.

The choice of generic, diagnosis-specific, or diagnosis-considered measures of severity of illness depends mainly on the hypotheses and populations of interest. Generic measures reflect basic physiological functioning and can usually be collected on all types of populations. Diagnosis-specific measures are useful when only one, or at most several, conditions are being studied. When data on a large number of patients with many disparate conditions are being collected, diagnosis-considered severity rating systems may be most appropriate. It is important to note that more than one type of severity measure can be used in a study, and different measures may add different types of information to the analysis.

The Relationship between Severity of Illness and Comorbidity

Although often considered separately from severity measures in the literature, comorbidity is a component of the patient's overall severity of illness. Defining the concepts of *severity of disease, comorbidity*, and *severity of illness* by referring to the literature is a confusing task, since many measures use the terms interchangeably. These definitions can be clarified by outlining the relationship of these constructs to each other.

Severity of disease. Severity of disease usually refers to the severity and importance of a particular diagnosis (often the principal diagnosis) to the patient's risk of an untoward outcome, regardless of a patient's other health conditions. For example, a patient with a principal diagnosis of cancer may be staged from I to IV, with I being less severe (representing local disease) and IV being the most severe (representing widely metastatic spread). Diagnosis-specific measures are similarly defined and measure the severity and importance of the principal diagnosis:

$$\textbf{Severity of disease} = f \begin{cases} \text{Importance of the principal diagnosis} \\ \text{Severity of the principal diagnosis} \end{cases}$$

Comorbidity. The term *comorbid conditions* refers to one or more additional diagnoses for a patient, not the principal diagnosis that brought the patient into the health care system. (Comorbidity is discussed at greater length in the next chapter.) A measure of comorbidity implicitly or explicitly weights the severity of each individual diagnosis and the importance of each diagnosis to the overall level of comorbidity for the patient. For example, the Charlson Comorbidity Index sums scores for approximately 20 diseases, ranging from stroke to liver disease (Charlson et al., 1987). Diseases not included in calculating the score are implicitly weighted zero. Each disease receives a score from 1 to 6, representing the importance of the disease to the overall level of comorbidity and relative risk of death. For example, congestive heart failure is weighted as 1, while AIDS or metastatic cancer is weighted as 6. In addition, several diseases have weights that explicitly incorporate their severity. Mild liver disease receives a weight of 1, while moderate or severe liver disease is weighted 3.

$$\textbf{Comorbidity} = f \begin{cases} \text{Importance of each secondary diagnosis} \\ \text{Severity of each secondary diagnosis} \end{cases}$$

Severity of illness. Information about the severity of all a patient's diagnoses can be combined to get a score for a particular patient's overall level of illness. Consequently, overall severity of illness is a function of both the severity of disease and comorbidity. Similar to comorbidity indices, these measures weight both the severity of each diagnosis and the importance of each diagnosis to the overall level of illness for the patient. Diagnosis-considered measures of severity aggregate information using this approach. However, severity of illness can also be defined generically without reference to a specific diagnosis. These generic measures identify variables representing basic disorders of organ functioning and score these variables identically across all patients. The types of severity measures used in an individual study will depend on the underlying conceptual model and the research questions being asked.

$$\textbf{Overall severity of} \begin{cases} \text{Importance of the principal diagnosis} \\ \text{Severity of the principal diagnosis} \\ \text{Importance of each secondary diagnosis} \\ \text{Severity of each secondary diagnosis} \end{cases}$$

The Timing of Measurement

Ideally, information about the severity of illness should be collected at two time points (see Figure 6–2).

1. prior to symptom onset
2. after symptom onset but prior to intervention (at presentation)

Measurement of the patient's burden of disease prior to symptom onset may be as important as measurement of severity after the onset of symptoms. For example, one patient may be debilitated and living in a nursing home, while another patient is completely independent and lives alone in his or her own home. Both patients have identical strokes and become paralyzed on the right side of their bodies. The first patient has a substantially higher probability of a poor outcome. Failure to account for this fact may jeopardize the ability to examine the treatment effect. Information on these patients' levels of functioning prior to the onset of their acute strokes is essential to predicting their long-term outcomes. Often this information will be collected retrospectively (e.g., hospitalized patients may be interviewed about their level of functioning prior to the onset of symptoms).

Many severity measures incorporate information about the patient after the intervention of interest already has been implemented. Depending on the study, this may completely invalidate the use of a measure. In all cases, such use is substantially problematic. In particular, if an investigator believes that any components of the severity measure might be affected by the intervention, a different measure should be used, or the time points for data collection should be restricted to the time prior to the intervention. If the original measure were naively used to adjust for severity of illness, it could easily adjust away the effects of the intervention! Changes in a patient's condition after the intervention has been implemented should be identified as complications, not comorbidities or other components of severity, and should be dealt with separately. Complications are outcome events that are specific to an intervention or diagnosis. Complications should never be adjusted for in the analysis. This issue is discussed more fully in the following chapter.

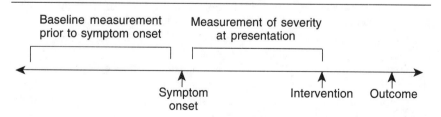

Figure 6–2 Timeline for Measurement of Severity of Illness

The timing of measurement is particularly easy to illustrate for baseline measures of the outcome variable. These measures differ from the final measures of outcome only in the timing of data collection. For example, suppose the outcome of interest is physical functioning at discharge for patients who present to the hospital with acute stroke. Information can be collected on the patients' level of functioning at admission to the hospital and prior to the onset of symptoms. These values can be used to adjust for the potentially confounding effects of differences in both the severity of the initial stroke and differences in the baseline levels of functioning prior to the stroke.

Including Severity Measures in Conceptual Models

There are several reasons to incorporate severity of illness measures explicitly into the conceptual models driving outcomes research. These include adjusting for selection bias, improving the ability of the model to predict outcomes, and forming a basis for subgroup analyses. The following sections examine the beneficial consequences of including these measures in the initial conceptualization. After the data have been collected, statistical testing of these models can incorporate information about the initial severity of illness and substantially increase the validity and credibility of the results.

Identification of Selection Bias

In most outcomes research, groups are not randomly allocated to the intervention of interest. This creates the potential for substantial selection bias. If sicker patients are less likely to receive the intervention, comparison of the intervention and nonintervention groups is likely to show a favorable outcome for patients who receive the intervention. This favorable outcome is not due to the effect of the intervention but is the result of a healthier set of patients in the intervention group. Two criteria must be met in order for selection bias to occur (see Figure 6–3). First, severity of illness must be related to the outcome of interest. Second, the severity of illness must influence which patients receive the intervention.

One practical way to identify components of severity important in creating potential selection bias is to look at the indications for the intervention. For example, suppose the outcomes research question is whether coronary angioplasty is effective in reducing mortality in a group of patients with angina. The comparison group is composed of patients with angina who do not receive angioplasty. If the severity of coronary occlusion is an indicator for angioplasty and is related to eventual mortality, then it is likely that substantial selection bias will occur if the severity of coronary occlusion is not included in the analysis.

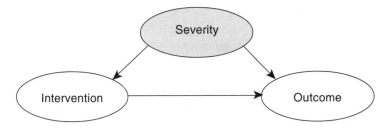

Figure 6–3 Identification of Selection Bias

The direction of the resulting bias cannot always be predicted in advance. For example, if sicker patients are more likely to receive the intervention, the intervention group may do more poorly than the comparison group, but this is due to the initial poor health of patients receiving the intervention, not the intervention itself. Because the direction of the bias cannot always be predicted, it is important to include severity measures in conceptual models of outcomes research and to use these models in developing the statistical methods for final analysis.

Independent Predictors of Outcome

Even when there is no evidence of biased selection, severity of illness measures are often believed to be important factors predicting the outcome. In this case, severity of illness is strongly related to outcome (see Figure 6–4) but is not related to whether or not a patient ends up in the intervention group. Although there is no risk of biased conclusions, including severity in the statistical models may substantially improve their fit and, consequently, improve the precision of the estimates for the impact of the intervention. Here, the benefit of measuring severity is indirect but, again, argues for including these measures in conceptual and statistical models of the outcome.

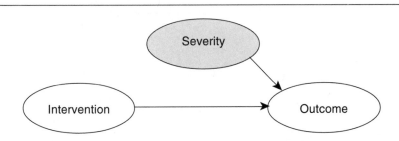

Figure 6–4 Independent Predictors of Outcome

Subgroup Analysis

The relationship between the intervention and outcome may differ depending on the severity of the illness. Subgroups of patients with more or less severe disease may respond differently to an intervention. In this case, severity may or may not be directly related to the intervention or the outcome. However, the impact of the intervention is substantially different depending on the initial levels of severity of the patients. The impact of severity on the relationship between the intervention and outcome is shown in Figure 6–5. When this situation occurs, subgroups should be analyzed separately, or appropriate statistical interaction terms should be included in the model.

HOW DO OUTCOMES RESEARCHERS CHOOSE A SEVERITY MEASURE?

A variety of tools are available for evaluating measures of severity of illness. The list of criteria shown in Exhibit 6–2 should help investigators choose the most appropriate measures.

Included Domains

The investigator must make sure that all relevant domains of health are included. It is unlikely that all important domains will be incorporated into a single measure of severity. Consequently, several measures are often used to cover all domains considered important for risk adjustment. For example, an investigator might consider initial levels of physical functioning, emotional functioning, and cognition relevant to the outcome of interest. Separate measures of each domain could be chosen, or measures that combine one or more domains could be used.

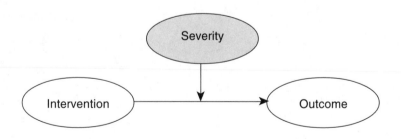

Figure 6–5 Subgroup analysis

Exhibit 6–2 Criteria for Choosing a Severity Measure

- Included domains
- Reliability
- Validity
  1. Prognostic end point
  2. Population of interest
  3. Setting
  4. Data collection method
  5. Timing of measurement

The relevant domains can be chosen by one of several methods, including:

- **Iezzoni's test (Iezzoni, 1994) of medical meaningfulness:** Is the domain linked to the outcome of interest?
- **Test of influence:** Does the domain directly or indirectly affect the outcome based on a specific conceptual model?

The second method explicitly incorporates the concept of subgroup analysis described earlier. In this case, the domain of interest may not be directly related to the outcome, but if it is indirectly related (i.e., affects the patient's response to treatment), then it should be measured and included in the analysis on that basis.

Reliability

Measures of severity must be reliable (i.e., dependable), particularly given the controversy over the effectiveness of statistical risk adjustment strategies. Since unreliable measures cannot be valid, the entire validity of an outcomes study could be questioned if unreliable measures are used. (See Chapter 9 for a more complete discussion of reliability.)

Validity

An important, but often overlooked, question to ask before using any severity measure is this: how was the measure validated? (See Chapter 9 for a more complete discussion of validity.) Most measures of severity are validated by showing that they predict an outcome measure of interest (e.g., mortality) under certain conditions. Therefore, some severity measures explicitly incorporate prognosis into their construction. However, it is important to note that this validity is conditional. A particular severity measure is valid only in situations with similar characteristics. For example, a measure validated by predicting in-hospital mortality for adult patients admitted to an intensive care unit can be considered reasonably valid for use in a similar inpatient population but should definitely not be assumed valid for use in a study examining the functional status of children with rheumatoid arthritis in an outpatient setting. The more closely an investigator's study resembles the circumstances where a measure was validated, the more likely it is that the measure will be successful in capturing the important components of severity.

The validity of a severity measure is particularly important if it does not "work." That is, if a severity measure utilized in an outcomes analysis cannot be shown to be statistically related to the outcome of interest or to identify important subgroups for analysis, then the fundamental validity of a measure should be questioned. It is indeed possible that the measure has never been validated for that purpose. To avoid this unfortunate situation, a researcher should closely examine the circumstances under which a measure has been validated and consider the consequences of not meeting one of the five main validation criteria in the study: prognostic end point, population of interest, setting, data collection method, and timing of measurement (see Exhibit 6–2).

Prognostic End Point

Severity measures are considered valid if they can be shown to predict strongly the outcome of interest. This validation process meets the earlier definition of severity (an estimate of the risk of an untoward outcome). Most measures of severity have been validated for only one outcome (usually in-hospital mortality). However, clinical outcomes are not the only outcomes of interest in today's health care market. Wood, Ament, and Kobrinski (1981) use three categories to classify the end point used to validate severity measures (i.e., the prognostic end point):

1. medical meaningfulness (e.g., death, nursing home placement, functional status)
2. economic meaningfulness (e.g., resource consumption)
3. administrative meaningfulness (e.g., length of stay)

A severity measure should be selected that has been validated against the outcome of interest in the current study. There is some overlap; some measures have been validated for more than one type of prognostic end point, and this makes them particularly useful in studies examining more than one type of outcome.

Population of Interest

There are numerous populations of interest in outcomes research. These include children, young adults, older adults, psychiatric patients, patients with end-stage renal disease; the list is essentially endless. Unfortunately, a severity measure may work differently in different populations, and it may be difficult to find a measure validated on a population identical to the proposed population. Some compromises are better than others. If an investigator plans to study a population of hospitalized adult patients with chronic renal disease, it is reasonable to use a measure of severity validated on all hospitalized adult patients, although it would be best to combine this measure of severity with other markers known to be important in chronic renal disease (e.g., creatinine levels). It is unlikely that a measure of severity developed for psychiatric patients would be useful.

Setting

The number of settings in which patients receive care is rapidly expanding. For example, frail, older adults are cared for at home, in nursing homes, in adult day-care centers, in assisted living centers, and so forth. As a result, it is unlikely that a severity measure for frail older adults will have been validated in every setting. As before, it is important to make conscious compromises to the validity of a measure by considering this issue explicitly before a method is chosen. In particular, if a measure has been found to be valid in several settings similar to the one of interest, it is a good choice for use in a setting where no validated measures are available.

Data Collection Method

Dramatic differences can be apparent in information quality, quantity, validity, and reliability for the different types of data used in outcomes research. There are currently three main types of data: administrative databases, medical records, and patient surveys. Each type has different costs and benefits. There are certain outcomes (e.g., pain) that are extraordinarily difficult to collect in a reliable and valid manner from administrative databases or medical records. The solution (albeit a more expensive one) is to ask the patient directly. However, other types of data may only be available from medical records, such as the administration and timing of various therapies or medications, while data on hospital costs may be available only from administrative records.

Unfortunately, most severity measures have been developed for use with medical records or administrative databases. Substantially less effort has gone into measuring the severity of illness using information obtained directly from patients, whereas many outcome measures have been derived for use in direct patient surveys. It is important to remember that baseline measures of the outcomes of interest can almost always be used to measure the initial severity of illness. The usefulness of this approach has probably contributed to the paucity of severity measures developed for use in patient surveys. Information from different sources can be combined to measure severity. Measuring severity by more than one method improves the probability of identifying a successful measure, particularly if all five criteria for validity are not met for each individual measure.

Timing of Measurement

As discussed earlier, the timing of data collection for severity measures can have profound consequences for the results. The most important issue is to relate the timing of data collection for severity to the intervention of interest. Ideally, information on severity should be collected just prior to the application of the intervention. Often, some overlap is unavoidable, but the consequences of confounding the severity of the initial illness with the effects of the intervention should be considered explicitly. Unfortunately, several widely used measures of severity for hospitalized patients collect data from the entire hospitalization. The timing of data collection for potential severity measures should be carefully examined and linked to the conceptual model showing the relationship between the intervention and the outcome. If a potential severity measure utilizes data collected after the application of the intervention, another measure should be chosen.

Components of Variable Construction

Information on variable construction is necessary for several reasons, including relating the severity measure to the conceptual model of the outcome and identifying issues important for subsequent statistical analysis. Three components of variable construction are described, including the level of categorization of the variables, the scale of the measurement, and the range of possible scores (Exhibit 6–3).

Level of Categorization

As discussed earlier, severity measures can be categorized as generic, diagnosis specific, or diagnosis considered. The choice of one or more measures depends mainly on the conceptual model and populations of interest. If the population

---

Exhibit 6–3 Components of Variable Construction

- Level of categorization
- Measurement scale
- Range of scores

under study can be defined by a principal diagnosis, it is reasonable to focus on a diagnosis-specific measure, perhaps along with a generic measure to capture a broad array of organ dysfunction or an additional measure of comorbidity (see the following chapter). If the population includes patients with many different principal diagnoses, a generic measure may become the primary measure of severity, or another measure that combines a wide variety of disease-specific scores may be useful (i.e., a diagnosis-considered measure). Generic measures are particularly useful when information is not available on the severity of individual diagnoses.

Comorbidity measures are often collected in addition to measures of severity of illness. These comorbidity measures may be less useful in studies using a diagnosis-considered severity measure. This is not because the concept of comorbidity has been lost, but only because the broader based measures of severity of illness incorporate information about comorbid conditions into their construction.

Measurement Scale

The advantages and disadvantages of continuous versus categorical measures of severity should be considered. These issues are discussed more fully in Chapter 9. Continuous (i.e., interval) data are almost always preferred from a statistical standpoint. Statistical treatment of categorical measures (e.g., nominal or ordinal) may be more complex, and these measures may provide less detail about the precise level of severity of initial illness.

Range of Scores

The range of scores is most important for categorical measures of severity, as each additional category slightly lowers the statistical power of a study. For example, diagnosis-related groups (DRGs) use almost 500 separate categories to classify patients. This number of categories is clearly manageable from a statistical standpoint only if the sample size is in the tens of thousands. Continuous (interval) measures do not have this problem, although they may have other types of problems, such as the presence of influential outliers.

WHAT SPECIFIC MEASURES ARE AVAILABLE TO OUTCOMES RESEARCHERS?

The number of severity measures in the literature has expanded dramatically over the last two decades. Many of these measures have been through several revisions. It would be impossible to provide a detailed analysis of all of these severity measurement systems within the scope of this chapter. The tools developed in the preceding section provide a useful starting point for a brief analysis of several representative measures.

Severity Measures

Several measures were chosen to represent important aspects of severity measurement, including the Acute Physiology, Age and Chronic Health Evaluation (APACHE), Computerized Severity Index (CSI), DRGs, Disease Staging (DS), and Medisgroups. These measures were included because they have demonstrated adequate reliability and validity over time. Table 6–1 examines the reliability, validity, and variable construction for these measures. All were developed for use on hospitalized patients; the development of measures for other patient populations has proceeded more slowly.

APACHE

Intensive care units (ICUs) admit patients with a wide variety of diagnoses, and these patients account for a substantial portion of hospital expenditures (Knaus, Draper, & Wagner, 1983). In most cases, patients are admitted to ICUs because of broad-based organ dysfunction (e.g., cardiovascular or respiratory collapse), not because of their primary diagnosis. The original APACHE scoring system was developed to predict the risk of death in these patients and consisted of two parts: an acute physiology score (APS) and a chronic health evaluation (CHE) score. Thirty-three variables comprised the APS and represented measures of generic physiological functioning during the first 32 hours (e.g., heart rate, respiratory rate, urine output, hematocrit). Each variable was weighted from 1 to 4 based on a literature review and the consensus from a panel of physicians, and all variables were totaled to get a final APS value. The CHE was a four-category scale (from A to D) representing physiological reserve. Consequently, each patient was assigned a category (such as 20-A) that combined information regarding both of these measures. Due to criticism of the large number of variables and time allowed for data collection, the APACHE scoring system was subsequently revised (Wong & Knaus, 1991).

The APACHE II was developed in 1985 and was explicitly based on statistical modeling of in-hospital mortality (Table 6–1). The time period during which data were collected was reduced to the first 24 hours. The number of APS variables was reduced from 33 to 12, and the threshold and weights of variables were modified. Surgical procedures and age were incorporated into the score, and chronic health points were assigned only if the patient had a history of severe organ system insufficiency or was immunocompromised. The subsequent APACHE II summed the values from three parts: APS points, age points, and chronic health points.

Table 6–1 Reliability, Validity, and Variable Construction for Severity of Illness Measures

	APACHE II	DRG	CSI	DS (Clinical)	DS (Scale)	Medisgroups (Original)
Reliability	Gamma = .925 Tau-B = .837*	ICC = .899*	Kappa = .88†	Not available	ICC = .708†	Gamma = .92 Tau-B = .78*
Validity						
Relevant end point	In-hospital mortality	Total charges, LOS	Treatment difficulty (length of stay)	Organ system involvement, risk of complications	In-hospital mortality, LOS total charges	In-hospital mortality and morbidity
Patient population	Adult patients	Patients	Patients	Patients	Patients	Patients
Setting	Hospital intensive care unit	Hospital	Hospital	Multiple settings	Hospital	Hospital
Data requirements	Medical record review	Discharge abstract	Medical record review	Medical record review	Discharge abstract	Medical record review
Timing of measurement	Worst value during first 24 hours	Entire hospitalization	Any time point	Any time period	Entire hospitalization	Worst value over first 48 hours
Variable construction						
Level of categorization	Generic	Procedure- or diagnosis-specific	Combines disease-specific scores	Diagnosis-specific	Combines disease-specific scores	Generic
Measurement scale	Interval	Nominal	Ordinal	Ordinal	Interval	Ordinal
Range of scores	Score: 0–71	467 categories	Scores: 1–4 for each of 820 disease groups and overall	Stages: 1.0–3.0 for each of 420 diagnoses	Relative weights with the average set equal to 100 for each scale	Score: 0–4

Notes:
LOS = length of stay, ICC = intraclass correlation coefficient.
*See Thomas and Ashcraft (1989).
†See Horn et al. (1991).

Recently, a second revision (Knaus et al., 1991) was developed (APACHE III) to improve the predictive value of the scoring system and to incorporate information about ICU organization and management that may contribute to hospital care.

DRGs

In the late 1970s, there was increasing interest in containing the growth in health care costs. In order to compare costs across hospitals, measures of hospital case mix were needed. DRGs were developed to define hospital case mix by grouping patients with similar clinical attributes and output utilization patterns (Fetter et al., 1980). Length of stay was considered to be the primary utilization pattern of interest. DRGs classified each patient into a major group based on the patient's primary diagnosis. Other variables, such as surgical procedures and the patient's age, were used to refine the classification so that patients with similar lengths of stay were grouped together. The result was 383 DRGs that were medically meaningful and that grouped patients with respect to a major indicator of output utilization (length of stay).

In 1983, Medicare began paying hospitals based on an expanded set of 467 DRG categories (Table 6–1; Vladeck, 1984). As a result of their widespread use as a payment mechanism and criticism regarding the relative paucity of information about severity of illness, DRGs recently have been refined through the addition of information regarding secondary diagnoses (Freeman et al., 1995). Nevertheless, since DRGs use information from the entire hospitalization, they may represent the effects of therapeutic interventions in addition to the underlying severity of the initial illness. Their use as a risk adjustment tool remains limited, although their value for reimbursement purposes makes them an important focal point for the development of more refined measures of severity of illness.

Computerized Severity Index

After criticism of DRGs' ability to classify severity of illness, the CSI was developed as an alternative (Table 6–1; Horn et al., 1991). The CSI is based on the International Classification of Diseases, Ninth Revision (ICD-9) coding system (U.S. Public Health Service, 1980), which indicates the existence of disease by assigning a code to a specific diagnosis. The CSI extends the ICD-9 coding system by incorporating diagnosis-specific information about disease severity. The definition of severity used for developing the CSI was treatment difficulty (proxied by length of stay) due to the extent of and interactions with a patient's diagnoses (Iezzoni et al., 1992). The CSI uses explicit criteria to assign a severity level from 1 to 4 for each diagnosis. This system also combines information about diagnoses using disease-specific weighting rules and assigns an overall patient severity level from 1 to 4.

Disease Staging

The original clinical version of disease staging is based on a purely conceptual model of disease severity (Gonnella, et al., 1984). Its unique conceptual basis makes it worth a brief examination, although the reliability and validity of the original version have not been reported in detail (Table 6–1). In disease staging, each diagnosis represents a disease (not a symptom or physical abnormality) that is conceptualized based on the organ system involved (e.g., cardiovascular) and the etiology (e.g., degenerative). A level of severity (from 1.0 to 3.0, with 4.0 representing death) is assigned to each disease based on the degree of complications and generalized systemic involvement. A panel of medical consultants specified disease-specific staging criteria for approximately 400 diseases.

A computerized version of disease staging was developed empirically using information from the entire hospitalization (Table 6–1; Markson et al., 1991). This version incorporates information regarding the stage of each of a patient's diseases, and other patient characteristics. Three different scales are produced for each patient, based on separate predictions of in-hospital mortality, length of stay, and in-hospital charges. As mentioned earlier, the use of information from the entire hospitalization may confound the effects of therapeutic interventions with the underlying severity of the initial illness and limits the broad applicability of this measure for risk adjustment.

Medisgroups

Medisgroups is an instrument that classifies patients into one of five severity groupings at admission based on relative degree of organ failure (Table 6–1; Brewster et al., 1985). Patients are initially categorized by the reason for admission, although this categorization is not used in the final severity grouping. The assignment of a patient to a severity group is based on key clinical findings (KCFs), which are objective indicators of abnormal physiology (e.g., electrocardiogram, chest X-ray, respiratory rate). The level of each KCF receives a score from 1 to 4, and the most severe KCF determines the patient's severity grouping (even if it is unrelated to the reason for admission).

Domains of Health

Table 6–2 identifies the domains of health included in each of these severity measures. These domains were described in detail in Chapter 2 and may include physical functioning, social functioning, emotional functioning, cognitive functioning, symptoms (or pain), and vitality. Each severity measure incorporates information about the patient's physical functioning. The APACHE II measure

Table 6–2 Domains of Health Included in Severity of Illness Measures

Domains of Health	APACHE II	DRG	CSI	DS (Clinical)	DS (Scale)	Medisgroups (Original)
Physical function	+	±	+	+	+	+
Emotional function	−	±	−	−	−	−
Cognitive function	+	±	±	±	±	+
Social function	−	−	−	−	−	−
Symptoms	−	−	+	±	±	−
Vitality	−	−	−	−	−	−

Notes:
+ = Domain included in the severity measure.
− = Domain not included in the severity measure
± = Domain may be included in the severity measure depending on the primary diagnosis.

---

focuses almost exclusively on physical functioning but includes a crude measure of cognitive function (the Glasgow Coma Score). Since DRGs assign patients to a primary diagnostic category, these categories include broad groupings of mental disorders and diseases of the nervous system. This allows identification of the domain for a patient's major diagnosis, although other domains of interest are not identified. The CSI is based on diagnosis-specific information, which incorporates information regarding both physical functioning and symptoms, and may include a measure of cognitive status (depending on the diagnosis). Disease staging scores focus mainly on physical functioning, although crude measures of cognitive function or symptoms may be incorporated (e.g., chest pain for myocardial infarction patients). The domains covered by the Medisgroups score are similar to the APACHE II; almost all the KCFs cover physical functioning, although coma or stupor on neurological examination is assigned to Severity Group 3. None of the measures covers the domains of social function or vitality, and few measures cover more than two to three domains of health. If the conceptual model of the outcome includes domains not covered by the severity measure under consideration, additional measures will be needed to adjust for the initial severity of these other domains of health (see Chapters 2, 3, and 8).

CONCLUSION

This chapter has examined the conceptual and methodological issues involved in measuring severity of illness in outcomes research. Many severity of illness measures have been developed, but all have limitations. Most focus on physiological functioning to the exclusion of other domains of health. Others have not been adequately tested for reliability and validity across a wide range of settings. Few measures are available for non-hospital settings such as nursing homes or ambulatory care clinics. A recent comparison of severity-adjusted mortality rates suggested that judgments about hospital performance can vary depending on which severity measure was used (Iezzoni et al., 1996). Consequently, compromises must often be made when conducting an outcomes research study. When choosing a set of severity measures, the goal should be to make explicit and conscious compromises (when necessary) to the data collection and analytic strategy based on a well-conceived conceptual model. This conceptual model should explicitly link the intervention of interest to the outcome, incorporate information regarding all important and related domains of initial health, and set a specific timeline for retrospective or prospective data collection that will not confound the relationship of severity of illness with the complications of the intervention. This approach allows a closer approximation to answer the fundamental question of outcomes research: is the patient truly better off as a result of our intervention?

REFERENCES

Aronow, D.B. (1988). Severity of illness measurement: Applications in quality assurance and utilization review. *Medical Care Review, 45*, 339–366.

Brewster, A.C., Karlin, B.G., Hyde, A.A., Jacobs, C.M., Bradbury, R.C., & Chae, Y.M. (1985). MEDISGRPS. A clinically based approach to classifying hospital patients at admission. *Inquiry, 22*, 377–387.

Charlson, M.E., Pompei, P., Ales, K.L., & MacKenzie, C.R. (1987). A new method of classifying prognostic comorbidity in longitudinal studies: Development and validation. *Journal of Chronic Disease, 40*(5), 373–383.

Fetter, R.B, Shin, Y., Freeman, J.L., Averill, R.F., & Thompson, J.D. (1980). Case mix definition by diagnosis-related groups. *Medical Care, 18*, 1–53.

Freeman, J.L., Fetter, R.B., Park, H., Schneider, K.C., Lichtenstein, J.L., Hughes, J.S., Bauman, W.A., Duncan, C.C., Freeman, D.H., & Palmer, G.R. (1995). Diagnosis-related group refinement with diagnosis- and procedure-specific comorbidities and complications. *Medical Care, 33*, 806–827.

Gonnella, J.S., Hornbrook, M.C., & Louis, D.Z. (1984). Staging of disease: A case-mix measurement. *JAMA, 251*(5), 637–644.

Green J., Winfield, N., Sharkey, P., & Passman, L.J. (1990). The importance of severity of illness in assessing hospital mortality. *JAMA, 263*, 241–246.

Horn, S.D., Sharkey, P.D., Buckle, J.M., et al. (1991). The relationship between severity of illness and hospital length of stay and mortality. *Medical Care, 29*, 305–317.

Iezzoni, L. (Ed.). (1994). *Risk adjustment for measuring health outcomes.* Ann Arbor, MI: Health Administration Press.

Iezzoni, L.I., Ash, A.S., Coffman, G.A., & Moskowitz, M.A. (1992). Predicting in-hospital mortality: A comparison of severity measurement approaches. *Medical Care, 30*, 347–359.

Iezzoni, L.I., Ash, A.S., Schwartz, M., Daley, J., Hughes, J.S., & Mackiernan, Y.D. (1996). Judging hospitals by severity-adjusted mortality rates: The influence of the severity-adjustment method. *American Journal of Public Health, 86*: 1,379–1,387.

30262.

Knaus, W.A., Draper, E.A., & Wagner, D.P. (1983). Toward quality review in intensive care: The APACHE system. *Quality Review Bulletin, 9*(7), 196–204.

Knaus, W.A., Draper, E.A., Wagner, D.P., & Zimmerman, J.E. (1985). APACHE II: A severity of disease classification system. *Critical Care Medicine, 13*(10): 818–829.

Knaus, W.A., Wagner, D.P., Draper, E.A., Zimmerman, J.E., Bergner, M., Bastos, P.G., Sirio, C.A., Murphy, D.J., Lotring, T., Damiano, A.D., Harrell, F.E. (1991). The APACHE III prognostic system: Risk prediction of hospital mortality for critically ill hospitalized adults. *Chest 100*, 1,619–1,636.

Markson, L.E., Nash, D.B., Louis, D.Z., & Gonnella, J.S. (1991). Clinical outcomes management and disease staging. *Evaluation and the Health Professions, 14*(2), 201–227.

Pompei, P., Charlson, M., Ales, K., MacKenzie, C., & Norton, M. (1991). Relating patient characteristics at the time of admission to outcomes of hospitalization. *Journal of Clinical Epidemiology, 44*(10), 1,063–1,069.

Thomas, J.W., Ashcraft, M.L.F. (1989). Measuring severity of illness: A comparison of interrater reliability among severity methodologies. *Inquiry, 27*, 483–492.

U.S. Public Health Service, Health Care Financing Administration (1980). *The International Classification of Diseases, 9th Revision, Clinical Modification.* PHS 80-1260. Washington, DC: Author.

Vladeck, B.C. (1984). Medicare hospital payment by diagnosis related groups. *Annals of Internal Medicine, 100*, 576–591.

Wong, D.T., & Knaus, W.A. (1991). Predicting outcome in critical care: The current status of the APACHE prognostic scoring system. *Canadian Journal of Anesthesiology, 38*, 374–383.

Wood, W.R., Ament, R.P., & Kobrinski, E.J. (1981). A foundation for hospital case mix measurement. *Inquiry, 18*, 247–254.

7

Comorbidity

Nicole M. Nitz

WHAT IS COMORBIDITY?

Comorbid conditions are diseases other than the principal diagnosis that influence the outcome of treatment. Researchers can best understand what comorbidity is by examining its relationship to severity of illness. Person-specific severity of illness incorporates both the severity of the primary disease and the severity and number of comorbid conditions. The terms *severity of illness, severity of disease*, and *comorbidity* differ in the breadth of illness they delineate. *Severity of illness measures* assess the contribution to risk of the overall illness level, often as a sum of specific diseases. *Severity of disease* focuses on a specific condition, and *comorbidity* focuses on the contribution to risk of diseases other than the condition of primary interest.

The literature provides several conceptual frameworks for placing comorbidity in relation to severity of illness and complications. Greenfield et al. define comorbidity as "the state of health at admission apart from the primary diagnosis"

153

(1988, p. 2,253). Specifically, they relate the concept of comorbidity to those of severity of disease and complications by breaking down the assessment of health status for inpatients into these three constructs:

1. severity of the primary condition
2. severity of coexisting medical conditions and functional impairment due to these diseases or other diseases not documented in the medical history
3. conditions that arise during hospitalizations, either resulting from the hospitalization/treatment or unrelated

The first two of these constructs, severity of the primary condition and severity of coexisting medical conditions, constitute what was defined earlier as severity of illness and, ideally, are measured before treatment. The last construct, conditions that arise during hospitalization, concerns complications of the treatment.

Greenfield and Nelson (1992) differentiate comorbidity and severity of disease by describing the relationship of comorbid diseases to the disease of primary interest. First, comorbidity is measured as the aggregated effect of all the conditions the patient might have, excluding the primary condition of interest. Second, since comorbidities are secondary conditions, less information is available on them. Third, since by definition comorbidity is every illness *except* the condition of interest, the particular illnesses encompassed by this term will vary for each primary condition. Finally, the importance of a particular comorbid disease will differ depending on the primary condition of interest. Of these four criteria describing comorbidities, the second, stipulating that less data are available for comorbidities, will depend on the design of the study. The other three criteria provide a conceptual definition of comorbid diseases that is independent of the study design. Although investigators using historical (i.e., medical record) data might expect to find less data on the comorbidities than on the primary disease of interest, the amount of available data will often be comparable. Also, because historical data are generally derived from the records of clinicians and insurers rather than collected directly from patients and are heavily weighted to physical rather than psychological diagnoses, they will likely have an overall bias toward measuring comorbidities.

WHEN IS A CONDITION CONSIDERED COMORBID?

Investigators should be wary in adjusting for comorbidity, lest they inadvertently adjust for complications of the disease or treatment and, thus, adjust away the outcome of interest. It is important to differentiate between the constructs of comorbidity and complications. "Comorbidities, or coexisting diagnoses, are diseases unrelated in etiology or causality to the principal diagnosis," whereas complications are the "sequelae of the principal diagnosis" (or its treatment; Iezzoni, 1994, p. 52).

By expanding the above definitions of comorbidity and complication, coexisting conditions can be viewed in three ways: comorbidities, complications of disease, and complications of treatment. This expanded definition explicitly considers both the causality of the secondary condition and the time sequence of events. Here, *occurrence* of a disease means the time period of diagnosis, since knowing the true moment of the inception of the illness is often impossible, especially for chronic diseases.

Comorbidities

Comorbidities are conditions that are unrelated in etiology or causality to the principal diagnosis (e.g., cancer diagnosed after stroke). In terms of chronology, comorbid conditions may either precede, be concurrent with, or occur after the onset of the principal disease. Having a particular comorbid disease may increase (or decrease) the likelihood of a positive or negative outcome for the primary illness. In terms of measuring comorbid disease, one should control for comorbid diseases that occurred before the onset of the primary disease and before the treatment. Since the concept of a comorbid disease is rather arbitrarily defined by clinical logic, the decision to include in the measure conditions that occurred after the onset of the primary disease may depend on the clinical relevance of the comorbid condition to the primary disease.

Complications of the Disease

Complications of the disease are conditions that are directly causally/etiologically related to the principal disease itself. Specifically, we can view complications of the disease as disease-specific outcomes (see Chapter 3 for a further discussion of disease-specific outcomes). For example, in the case of diabetes and myocardial infarction, having the principal disease increases the likelihood that the secondary condition will develop. This implies that the complication must occur concurrent with or after the principal disease. Complications may also be related to comorbid diseases, especially when these diseases have a synergistic effect in increasing the vulnerability of the patient to infection. Disease complications may occur either before or after treatment is initiated, and when they occur will determine how the investigator should treat these complications. When an outcomes study is focused on hospitalizations, investigators reviewing hospital discharge records may identify complications of the disease that occur after admission. However, investigators should view complications of the disease that occur after the start of treatment as outcomes, rather than controlling for these factors. Preadmission complications of the primary disease may be incorporated into the measure of the severity of disease at admission. Including disease complications that occur *prior* to the intervention in a measure of disease severity and level of comorbidity should not bias the estimates of the effectiveness of the treatment. To the extent that treatment should address these disease complications, however, one would not want to adjust for their presence.

Complications of the Treatment

Complications of the treatment for the principal disease occur when a treatment for the principal disease causes the patient to suffer the secondary condition. We should be able to detect this type of complication by looking at differences in incidence rates for the condition across different types of treatment or no treatment. However, we do not want to control for treatment complications, since doing so will bias the estimate of treatment effect. A condition can be both a complication of disease and of the treatment, where the disease increases the likelihood of occurrence, but a particular treatment increases the likelihood even further than if the treatment had not been used. This type of complication must occur concurrent with or after the treatment and, therefore, after the diagnosis of the principal disease.

In practice, it may be impossible to differentiate between disease complications and treatment complications when they occur after the start of the treatment. Any complication that occurs after the beginning of the treatment should be regarded as an outcome of the treatment. One would not want to control for these post-treatment complications in the analysis, except with the complete understanding that doing so may bias the estimates of the effects of the treatment by controlling for the negative consequences of treatment.

While distinctions between complications and comorbidities can be made definitionally, the etiological relationship between diseases and particular episodes of illness may not always appear as clear-cut. Therefore, each study requires a clear conceptual model of which conditions will be considered complications as opposed to comorbidities to avoid inadvertently controlling for complications of the treatment. Controlling for comorbidities allows the investigator to attribute a better outcome to the treatment rather than to a healthier group of treatment subjects. On the other hand, controlling for complications of the treatment will make it appear that the treatment had a far better effect on outcomes than it really did. Including treatment complications in the comorbidity measure will increase the variance explained in the model but by explaining away the outcome (Shapiro et al., 1994).

WHY SHOULD WE MEASURE COMORBIDITY?

Differences between groups in the levels of comorbid disease may generate differences in the measured outcomes for these groups, confounding the effect of the treatment. As with the measurement of severity of illness, the primary reason for assessing comorbidity is to eliminate potential sources of observed variation in outcomes between groups to help to isolate the effects of treatment. However, it is more useful to measure comorbidity rather than overall severity of illness when the outcomes study focuses on a particular disease of primary interest. Comorbidity measures also help to establish the patient's usual health status before treatment. Because medical treatments rarely make patients healthier than they were before the onset of the episode of illness, the definition of *pretreatment state* provides an estimate for the maximum possible improvement in health available from the treatment. Finally, an investigator may want to include measures of comorbidity to enhance the credibility of the study. If others believe it to be an important predictor of the outcome, even in the absence of compelling evidence or theory, the omission of a comorbidity measure could call the results into question.

Comorbidity measures can influence estimates of the treatment effect in several ways. Concerns might address the effects of confounding and selection bias or the independent effect of comorbidity on the outcome, or one might wish to use comorbidity as the basis for a subgroup analysis.

Selection Bias

Comorbid conditions can influence the receipt and outcomes of treatment. Procedures that are appropriate for a person with few or no other illnesses may be inappropriate for a patient with other concurrent diseases. Clinicians and patients select treatments that are appropriate for the "package" of the primary illness and other existing conditions. *Selection bias* occurs when the group of patients receiving Treatment A are fundamentally different from the group of patients receiving Treatment B because one or more of the factors influencing the outcome also determined which treatment the patient received (Iezzoni et al., 1994). Along with the severity of the disease of primary interest, other illnesses that the patient has concurrent with the primary disease may also affect the outcomes of care as well as the type of treatment provided. The decision whether to include a measure of comorbidity and which one to use will depend on the treatment upon which the analysis focuses and the clinical logic of how treatments are selected.

Independent Predictors

Including measures of comorbidity may not only account for the effects of selection bias but also reveal the independent effects of other factors, controlling for comorbidity. Age often has been used as a substitute measure for comorbidity since it is easily measured, and, in clinical and sociological models, age is highly associated with a greater number and severity of illnesses. Age, however, is not a substitute for comorbidity because it has independent effects after controlling for comorbidity. Greenfield et al. (1987) found that when they controlled for the effect of comorbidity, there was still a difference by age in patterns of care for breast cancer, suggesting a possible age bias in treatment given to breast cancer patients.

Subgroup Analysis

The effect of the treatment on the outcome may differ with the level or types of comorbid conditions the patient has. This difference in effect has been to some extent recognized by the clinical logic used in selecting a treatment. Clinicians may recommend that patients with certain comorbid diseases not use a particular treatment because the treatment may not work as well or may be detrimental to people with those comorbid conditions. However, standard clinical treatment procedures do not always account for all possible conditions. The treatment effect might differ by the presence or level of comorbid conditions that were not considered to be clinically relevant to the choice of treatment or to the outcome.

HOW DO RESEARCHERS MEASURE COMORBIDITY AND CHOOSE A COMORBIDITY MEASURE?

General versus Condition-Specific Measures

In an ideal research world, investigators would be able to create a customized comorbidity measure for each primary diagnosis. However, given time and budget restrictions, this is not usually possible, so the investigator must resort to using a general measure created for use in another study. One must consider the practical losses incurred in using a general measure, especially the ability of the entire model to explain variances in the outcome. Additionally, using a general measure rather than a disease-specific measure will influence the size of the estimated effect of comorbidity on the outcome; the impact of comorbidity on the outcome, often measured by relative risks or regression coefficients, will vary depending on the measure used. A general measure may still be significantly related to the outcome, but the ability of the model to explain variance in the outcome may be lower than for a model using a disease-specific comorbidity measure. An alternative to using the general measure alone is for the investigator to use the general measure in combination with individual variables for other relevant diseases not addressed by the general measure. However, the sample size of the study population limits the number of independent variables one may include in the analysis because the sample size and the number of independent variables determine the degree of freedom.[1] Researchers subscribe to varying rules of thumb regarding the ratio of sample size to the number of independent variables, ranging from 5 to 20 observations per independent variable. The researcher should examine the adequacy of the study sample size relative to the number of independent variables included in the analysis. For example, if in lieu of using a single measure of comorbidity, the researcher uses 30 separate variables to represent 30 comorbid conditions, there are therefore 29 fewer degrees of freedom available for including other types of independent variables in the regression.

Disease of Primary Interest

Several critical issues should be considered in either choosing an already developed measure of comorbidity or creating a new measure. The study's primary disease or set of diseases will influence the choice of a measure for comorbid disease, since comorbid diseases are defined only in relation to the principal disease, and the types of data collected will differ depending on the primary disease. For example, in a study that compares outcomes among health care plans for a broad range of illnesses, from rheumatoid arthritis to stroke, the comorbidity measure appropriate to the outcomes for rheumatoid arthritis will likely be quite different from the comorbidity measure used in comparing outcomes for stroke. The diversity of diseases this type of study examines suggests using several comorbidity measures depending on which outcomes the investigator is analyzing. For example, investigators could employ a measure previously used to predict outpatient utilization in comparing outcomes for rheumatoid arthritis, but they should use a measure that predicts mortality when comparing stroke outcomes.

Reliability and Validity

Both reliability and validity are important in choosing a measure of comorbidity. The reliability (or reproducibility) of the measure limits the validity of the measure for the study; an instrument that does not consistently produce the same measurements for the same conditions is not likely to be measuring those conditions at all. Validity may be limited by the conditions under which the measure was validated. For example, a comorbidity measure for hospitalized adults used to predict mortality may be less valid for measuring the effect of comorbidity among young adults on health status. The younger population may be so healthy compared to the older, hospitalized population, that in the younger population, the measure cannot differentiate between sicker and healthier members; they might all get lumped into the "healthy" category, which is not very useful in an analysis.

Essential criteria for the suitability of comorbidity measures include the outcome, population, setting, and data source used to validate the measure. In examining these criteria, one may consider two questions:

1. Does the study match the criteria for which the measure was validated?
2. What are the consequences of not matching these criteria if the measure is chosen for this study?

Prognostic End Points

A basic reason to measure comorbid diseases is the assumption that they affect the study outcome, independently or by confounding the effect of the treatment or primary disease. The comorbidity measure should be expected to influence the outcome of primary concern. For example, an investigator might choose a comorbidity measure that was created to predict mortality. However, if the investigator is interested in an outcome other than mortality, a measure shown to predict mortality might not be the most appropriate one to use. This concern is especially relevant for ambulatory care, where death is an unlikely end point, and disability is more likely; a comorbidity measure created to predict mortality may not predict disability very well. Nonetheless, the end point used to establish the comorbidity measure need not necessarily be identical to the study outcome to explain some variance in the study outcome. Measures of comorbidity have been validated against many different outcomes, including mortality, outpatient services utilization, disability, and appropriateness of care (Charlson et al., 1987, 1994; Greenfield et al., 1987, 1988; Kahn et al., 1988; Parkerson, Broadhead, & Tse, 1993; Verbrugge, Lepkowski, & Imanaka, 1989). For example, the Charlson was created to predict mortality, whereas the ambulatory care groups (ACGs) were based on outpatient expected utilization.

A measure's inability to predict the relevant outcome in a given study may be interpreted in several ways. First, it may not measure the specific elements of comorbidity important to the outcome. Second, the specific comorbid conditions that were measured simply may not predict the outcome at all. Third, comorbidity may not predict the outcome in the study population due to unique characteristics of the study sample. The situation is clear if the measure chosen was validated against the same prognostic end point and in a similar population to those in the present study. Some external factor not accounted for in the model may affect the outcome itself. For example, if the study uses claims data from an insurance plan and hypothesizes that patients with greater comorbidity will use more mental health services, varying coverage limits on the number of mental health visits may make it difficult to assess the true size of the effect of comorbidity. In this case, the unmeasured confounding variables differed between the study population and the population used to validate the measure, and this is consistent with the third explanation above.

The measures of prognostic end points as well as the disease of primary interest will influence which comorbid conditions are weighted more heavily. In some measures, physical domains are weighted more heavily than cognitive or emotional domains. For example, if mortality is used as the end point, many cognitive and psychiatric conditions will be weighted lightly compared to physical conditions.

Unweighted Measures

The easiest method of measuring comorbid conditions would be simply to count the number of illnesses the patient has aside from the primary diagnosis. However, this simple summary approach has several weaknesses. First, by not explicitly assigning any weights, the actual weight each comorbid condition carries is the same; that is, this "unweighted" measure assumes that rheumatoid arthritis and stroke exert an equally important effect on the outcome, implicitly assigning each a weight of 1.0. This assumption may not be true. Second, this type of measure does not adjust for the severity of the comorbid conditions themselves. When we explicitly assign weights, we can give greater importance to cases in which the comorbid condition is more severe. (Severity adjustment was discussed at greater length in Chapter 6.) For example, if the comorbid condition is cancer, we can assign a larger weight to patients with a Stage IV diagnosis than to patients with a Stage I diagnosis.

Weighted Measures

The weights assigned to particular comorbid conditions will vary for different primary diagnoses. That is, a comorbid condition may have a greater influence on the outcome depending on the primary diagnosis. In addition, weights may be assigned not only to specific conditions but also to the severity of the comorbid conditions. In considering the weights assigned to each comorbid condition, the investigator should also examine the method used to combine the weighted comorbid disease into a score and decide whether this method is relevant to the disease of primary interest. For example, the Charlson Comorbidity Index (Charlson et al., 1987) uses an additive scale, assuming that the effect of combined diseases is equal to the added sum of their individual scores, weighted for severity. Counting the number of conditions may not be the appropriate method of aggregating the scale. Some diseases may have synergistic effects (i.e., combined with another disease, their effect is multiplicative rather than additive; Satariano, 1992).

Population

The population used to establish the relationship between comorbidity and outcome should resemble that addressed in the study at hand, since this population influences which conditions are weighted most heavily. There are two ways to calculate the weights: (1) for a population as a whole (e.g., the inpatient population in a hospital) and (2) for the specific population with the disease of interest (e.g., patients with diabetes). The weights calculated using a general population might be less applicable to a specific population. In particular, secondary conditions may have different implications for health relative to one disease compared to another. For example, physical diseases may be worse when cognitive impairments are present. In addition, measures that are validated among one population may not be sensitive to differences in levels of comorbid disease in another population (see Chapter 9 for a further discussion of the floor/ceiling effect in measurement).

Setting

Comorbidity measures have been validated in hospital and ambulatory care settings. The setting is closely tied to the population. The population in one setting may be fundamentally different from that in another, and setting can simply be viewed as another descriptor of the population.

Conditions or Diseases Included

A crucial issue in constructing a comorbidity measure is what diseases or conditions to include. Some measures limit the conditions to only those considered important (i.e., diseases not on the list have an implicit weight of 0). Other measures are comprehensive, assigning virtually all diagnostic codes some weight to incorporate them in the comorbidity scale whether or not they are relevant to the study outcome.

A structured list can make it easier to abstract from the medical records. One way to contain the length of such a list is to include only those with the largest effect on the outcome. In addition, such an explicit list also can account for differences in terminology used in medical records.

Measures of comorbidity may also include other risk factors that are not diseases, such as functional status, age, disease prognosis, or expected response to treatment (Charlson et al., 1987, 1994; Greenfield et al., 1987, 1988; Kahn et al., 1988; Parkerson et al., 1993). When measures include these other factors, the investigator will not be able to differentiate between the effect due to the comorbidity and the effect due to these factors. One should be careful not to include in the analysis these other factors if the comorbidity measure already includes them. For example, in using age-adjusted Charlson comorbidity scores, one should not also include age as a separate variable in the regression because the Charlson already accounts for age.

Timing of Measurement

Measuring the comorbid conditions prior to the treatment will ensure that treatment complications or post-treatment disease complications are not inadvertently included in the comorbidity measures. Inclusion of complications could make the treatment appear to be more beneficial than it really is. As discussed previously, it is difficult in practice to separate complications of treatment from complications of the disease that occur after the treatment. For example, a patient with diabetes enters the hospital for a myocardial infarction (MI) and has a stroke. It is unclear whether this is due to the treatment for the MI, or to the care received in the hospital after being admitted for the MI, or simply to the patient's illness. There are several plausible mechanisms by which hospital care could influence the development of a stroke. Therefore, the safest strategy is to exclude from the comorbidity measure any complication that occurs after the beginning of the treatment.

The duration and concurrence of the comorbid conditions should also be considered. Should the comorbidity measure only include conditions that are active? Some conditions may have long-term consequences for the patient's reaction to medical care. For example, previous hip fracture may make it more difficult for an older patient's subsequent hip fracture to heal. What kind of time frame will be used to determine whether or not the disease is still "active" if the data are not collected directly from the patient? The time frame used depends on clinical rationale and the availability of data. For example, a hip fracture that occurred 30 years ago may have less clinical relevance than one that occurred one year ago.

Data Sources

The choice of a comorbidity measure will determine the data source and vice versa. The investigator may use primary or secondary data or a combination of both. *Primary data collection* often involves surveys. Although new effort is required to abstract medical charts, one does not usually classify such data as primary. *Secondary data collection* may involve using data collected for another study or data from an administrative, medical records, or pharmacy database. The best source of data depends on the study and the particular biases of the data sources. Secondary data have the advantages of being relatively easy to obtain on a large number of subjects. However, external factors influence what type of data were originally collected, and these may affect the usefulness of these data for the study. *Prospective data collection* is almost always preferable but not always possible due to time or budgetary constraints. Prospective data permit collecting information that may otherwise not be available and collecting them in the level of detail sought. For example, the diagnosis of dementia may be inconsistently made, and rarely will clinicians provide enough information to stage it.

The reasons for recording data may affect its usefulness as secondary data. Most computerized or other secondary databases were not collected with outcomes research as a central or even peripheral concern. Their biases reflect the original reasons for collecting such data, the system used to record the data, and other pressures to change what data are recorded. Automated data usually mean less detailed information about lots of people; much information available from medical records may be lost. Investigators should be aware of where those gaps in knowledge occur in the databases they have selected, why they occur, and what biases may result from these gaps.

Medical Records Diagnoses

Although it seems that the medical records prepared by clinicians would be the most accurate method of determining other illness concurrent with the disease of primary interest, these data are not infallible. Clinicians vary in both the thoroughness of their recording and their diagnostic acumen. Errors of both omission and commission may occur. Some active diagnoses may not be recorded, and some inactive problems may be retained. Insurance limitations on which treatments are paid for may influence what the clinician records as the "official" record. A provider may choose a related problem or symptom that is secondary to the primary diagnosis. If a patient with depression had no coverage for mental health and is being prescribed antidepressants, a provider might record "sleep disturbance" as the diagnosis. The patient is probably having problems with sleep (since sleep disturbances are a symptom of the depression), so the visit will be covered (since antidepressants can also be prescribed for sleep). Medical records may also be difficult to abstract. For example, handwritten notes can cause significant abstraction error.

Administrative Computerized Diagnosis Records

Several issues associated with using administrative diagnosis records may affect the choice of a comorbidity measure. Standard terms for diseases and procedures are found in two common reference books, *The International Classification of Disease, Ninth Revision* (U.S. Public Health Service, 1980), referred to as ICD-9, and *The Physician's Current Procedural Terminology*, Fourth Edition (American Medical Association, 1994), referred to as CPT-4. First, the mapping of comorbidities to diagnostic ICD-9-clinical modification (CM) and *Current Procedural Terminology* (CPT-4) codes used in most databases is not necessarily very precise. How a comorbidity measure "maps" the clinical concept of the disease to the diagnostic and procedure codes may vary from measure to measure. Subtle distinctions may be lost or distorted. For example, should a comorbidity measure include ICD-9 codes for "minor depression" and "major depression" in the same way? A comparison of ICD-9-CM codes with clinical concepts of comorbidity found that some comorbid conditions cannot be precisely mapped to the ICD-9-CM or procedural codes (Romano et al., 1994).

Chronic or asymptomatic conditions may be less prevalent in computerized administrative databases. For example, for prostatectomy and cholecystectomy patients, hospital discharge data had less information on certain chronic conditions than did anesthesiologists' notes. As a result, these patients scored lower on the Charlson Comorbidity Index based on their discharge diagnoses but were judged to be a higher risk from the anesthesiologists' notes (Roos, Sharp, & Cohen, 1991). However, the exclusion of some types of information does not mean that the comorbidity measure will have less predictive power for the outcome. In this example, data from the hospital discharge notes and from the anesthesiology notes had similar predictive powers for 1-year mortality and 90-day readmission.

The number of secondary diagnoses allowed in the administrative database may be limited, either by budgetary constraints or by limitations on the number of diagnoses for which the clinic is paid. Again, this missing information may not have a large impact on the results of a study; the size of this effect depends on the comorbidity measure used, the outcome of interest, and the study question. For example, if the study hypothesizes that those with chronic diseases such as rheumatoid arthritis will have a higher mortality rate for hip fractures, the investigator will want to be sure that the computerized records are comprehensive enough to include chronic disease diagnoses when acute events are recorded.

Drug Prescription Data (from Medical Records or Computerized Database)

Many computerized insurance databases of prescriptions contain records of prescriptions filled by patients rather than prescriptions written by clinicians. Generally, this distinction may not be very important, but if one wants to use prescriptions as a proxy for illnesses, the prescribing behavior of clinicians is a more accurate reflection than only the subset of the prescriptions actually filled.

Prescription databases may also have a coverage bias; insurance claims or health maintenance organization (HMO) records may not reflect all prescriptions filled, particularly if the drug is either not covered by the insurance carrier or if the cost of the drug is less than the copayment the patient pays for prescription drugs. For example, some chronic diseases, such as arthritis, may be treated with non-prescription (over-the-counter) drugs, which would not be recorded in the database of filled prescriptions. Other drugs, such as penicillin (and even digoxin), are inexpensive enough that they would not be systematically found in the database. In addition, the types or brands of drugs included in the database may be limited to those on the formulary, particularly in the case of managed care pharmacies. Using prescription databases is even more problematic if there was a change in the formulary during the period of the study, so that a drug that was once covered is no longer covered or vice versa. Likewise, it pays to be alert to changes in Food and Drug Administration (FDA) regulations that permit drugs once sold only by prescription to be sold over-the-counter. For example, the change to over-the-counter status for medications used to treat yeast infections may have spurred a sudden drop in the number of prescriptions for these drugs, but this decline does not indicate a real decrease in the incidence of yeast infections.

WHAT ARE SOME EXAMPLES OF SPECIFIC COMORBIDITY MEASURES?

From among the range of available comorbidity measures, several existing measures were selected for illustrative purposes. One approach to measuring comorbidity involves using severity of illness or case-mix measures. To do so, the investigator would exclude the disease of primary interest when calculating the scores for the measures. In using measures in this manner, the investigator should carefully review the outcome against which the measure was validated and the population in which it was validated. Berlowitz, Rosen, and Moskowitz (1995) discuss several case-mix measures used in ambulatory care settings.

Measures such as the ACGs are actually case-mix measures that have been used as comorbidity measures by excluding the disease of primary interest when the investigators calculate the scores. Case-mix measures attempt to group patients by the risk (of mortality, of utilization) they share due to their illnesses, but the groups are not necessarily ranked. Severity of illness measures tend to rank patients based on their level of illness. Labeling a measure as a "comorbidity measure" is arbitrary and is based on how the researcher intends to use it and not necessarily how it was created. When used as comorbidity measures, the researcher may simply exclude the disease of primary interest from the data when calculating the measure. In this way, some of the measures discussed in this chapter, such as the Duke Severity of Illness Checklist, and the ACGs, could fit as easily into the previous chapter as severity of illness measures. Likewise, diagnosis-related groups (DRGs), discussed as a severity of illness measure in Chapter 6, could be used to assess comorbidity. Other case-mix or severity-of-illness measures can similarly be used to assess comorbidity as long as the disease of primary interest is first excluded before calculating scores for the measures.

As an alternative to using a preexisting comorbidity measure, each relevant comorbid disease can be used in the analysis separately. This approach allows more precise estimates of the specific effects of comorbid conditions, but it can generate a large number of independent variables. For example, if the investigator thinks that osteoarthritis has a particular effect on outcomes of hip fractures, he or she may put into the regression a variable representing whether or not the patient has osteoarthritis. The coefficient on this variable would tell the investigator the particular association between osteoarthritis and outcomes of hip fracture. However, this method can become very complex if many diseases are expected to influence the outcomes; the investigator may run into problems with the size of the study sample relative to the number of variables in the analyses.

Measures of comorbidity can be divided broadly into those intended for use in hospitalized populations and those created for use in ambulatory care settings.

Measures Developed for Use in Hospital Settings

Comorbidity Index

The Comorbidity Index (CI) was created to predict risk of mortality for hospitalized patients (Greenfield et al., 1988). The index consists of three subscales: initial severity of the comorbid conditions at admission, instability of comorbid conditions (complications) around time of admission, and functional status. The authors derived weights for this scale based on the Disease Staging System, a severity-of-illness measure (discussed further in Chapter 6). In the initial severity and instability subscales, weights for each comorbid condition are ordinal. This information is derived from medical records, where any condition that is mentioned at least twice by the physician is scored. The functional status subscale assigns points for functional status in 11 body systems, based on information from nurses' notes. These three subscales are combined into a single index that assigns subjects to one of four ordinal categories, ranging from a nondisease state to a condition of life-threatening illness. The number of categories has varied in different conceptions of the measure from 7 to 3. The CI was validated for an older adult population with primary diagnoses of breast, prostate, and colorectal cancers (Greenfield et al., 1987, 1988).

Charlson Comorbidity Index

The Charlson Comorbidity Index was originally created for use with medical chart abstracts to predict mortality for hospitalized patients (Charlson et al., 1987). It was then tested for its ability to predict 1-year mortality rates from comorbid disease in a population of women treated for breast cancer. Data about the comorbid conditions were collected from reviews of hospital records. Comorbid conditions are classified based on a clinical judgment of prognostic relevance; resolved conditions are excluded. The measure incorporates information about the severity of several common conditions. Weights for each disease were calculated from the adjusted relative risk of mortality associated with each disease. That is, diseases were weighted based on the ratio of the incidence rate of mortality for patients with the disease compared to the incidence rate of mortality for those without the disease. If patients with the disease were just as likely to die as patients without the disease, the relative risk of mortality for the disease would be 1.0. Weights for the relative risks were basically assigned according to a 3-point ordinal scale, with 1 point assigned to the conditions with the lowest relative risks and 3 points to those with the highest, but an exceptional rating of 6 was also used. Conditions with relative risks below 1.2 were dropped from the measure. Diseases with relative risks between 1.2 and 1.5 were assigned 1 point; diseases with relative risks of 1.5 to 2.5 were assigned 2 points; and diseases with relative risks of 2.5 to 6.0 were assigned 3 points; in addition, a small number of conditions with relative risks greater than 6 were assigned 6 points. In all, 19 conditions are included in the weighted measure. (See Table 7–1.)

The scores for each disease are then summed to create an index. The comorbidity index significantly predicts 1-year survival. Moreover, the model with the comorbidity index explains more variance in the outcome than the model with the disease entered individually. The comorbidity index has been refined further by combining information about the subject's age with the comorbid diseases in which each decade of age over 40 adds another point to the total comorbidity index score. The Charlson index worked as well as the Kaplan and Feinstein (Kaplan & Feinstein, 1974) method of classifying comorbid diseases in differentiating between patients with low and high levels of comorbidity and in explaining variance in mortality (Charlson et al., 1987, 1994). Additional studies have modified this instrument for use with (computerized) claims data by "mapping" the clinical disease definitions

Table 7–1 Conditions Included in the Charlson Comorbidity Index

Assigned Weight	Condition
1	Myocardial infarction
	Congestive heart failure
	Peripheral vascular disease
	Cerebrovascular disease
	Dementia
	Chronic pulmonary disease
	Connective tissue disease
	Ulcer disease
	Mild liver disease
	Diabetes
2	Hemiplegia
	Moderate or severe renal disease
	Diabetes with end organ damage
	Any tumor
	Leukemia
	Lymphoma
3	Moderate or severe liver disease
6	Metastatic solid tumor
	Acquired immunodeficiency syndrome (AIDS)

Source: Data from M.E. Charlson, P. Pompei, K.L., Ales, et al., A New Method of Classifying Prognostic Comorbidity in Longitudinal Studies: Development and Validation, *Journal of Chronic Diseases*, Vol. 40, pp. 373–383, © 1987.

to specific ICD-9-CM codes and for use with specific diseases of interest (Deyo, Cherkin, & Ciol, 1992; Romano, Roos, & Jollis, 1993a, 1993b; Roos et al., 1991).

Duke Severity of Illness Checklist

The Duke Severity of Illness Checklist was created to measure overall severity of illness but has been used as a measure of comorbidity by omitting the disease of primary interest in scoring the measure. For each comorbid disease, this instrument measures symptom level, complications, prognosis without treatment, and expected response to treatment. A severity score is then calculated for each disease by summing across these four domains. An overall score is created by summing across the severity scores for individual illnesses, with the highest weights assigned to the most severe diagnoses. This measure was validated for primary care adult outpatients ages 18 to 65. The measure was completed by the medical provider, by a checklist for the clinicians at the time of the patient encounter, or from medical charts. Some of the information required (prognosis without treatment and expected response to treatment) may be more difficult to derive from medical charts (Parkerson et al., 1993).

Kaplan and Feinstein

The Kaplan and Feinstein (1974) measure is a significant predictor of mortality from comorbid disease. It was originally validated as a comorbidity measure for mature-onset diabetes in an all-male Veterans Affairs (VA) hospital population. Diseases were categorized as diagnostically, prognostically, or pathogenically comorbid. Data were abstracted from medical charts. While weights for this measure were based on clinical judgment, it was equally able to differentiate between low- and high-risk groups for mortality from comorbid disease and explains as much variance as the empirically created Charlson Comorbidity Index (Charlson et al., 1987).

Measures Developed for Use in Ambulatory Care Settings

Chronic Disease Score

The Chronic Disease Score (CDS) was created in part to take advantage of the availability of large administrative databases available from health maintenance organization pharmacies (Von Korff, Wagner, & Saunders, 1992). The instrument was created as an indicator of chronic disease morbidity and health status in outpatients using drugs. This measure has been used as a measure of comorbidity by excluding the disease of interest from the measure. Because it does not include psychotropic drugs, it may also be used as originally constructed as a comorbidity measure when the disease of interest is psychological.[2] The CDS uses expert judgment to map the diseases most likely to be associated with certain classes of drugs. The measure includes 17 disease categories associated with drug classes (see Table 7–2).

The measure then assigns each of these classes of drugs a weight based on clinical judgments of the severity of these particular conditions relative to the other conditions, as well as the combination of classes of drugs being used. The weighted scores for each class of drugs are then summed to obtain a total CDS. This measure requires that the patient population have the same pharmacy data set. Unlike measures that are based on disease diagnoses, this measure is very susceptible to the economic and clinical environment from which the data are derived. Because this measure infers diagnoses from drug prescriptions, it is susceptible to technological changes in the types of drugs and medical therapies prescribed; this is especially a concern with regulatory changes that change the

Table 7–2 Medication Classes and Associated Chronic Disease Categories for the Chronic Disease Score

Disease Categories	Medication Classes
Heart disease	Anticoagulants, hemostatics
	Cardiac agents, angiotensin converting enzyme (ACE) inhibitors
	Diuretic loop
Respiratory illness	Isoproterenol
	Beta-adrenergic, miscellaneous
	Xanthine products
	Respiratory products including bronchodilators and mucolytics but excluding cromolyn
	Epinephrine
Asthma or rheumatism	Glucocorticoids
Rheumatoid arthritis	Gold Salts
Cancer	Antineoplastics
Parkinson's Disease	Larodopa®
Hypertension	Antihypertensives (except ACE inhibitors) or calcium channel blockers
	Beta blockers, diuretics
Diabetes	Insulin
	Oral hypoglycemics
Epilepsy	Anticonvulsants
Asthma or rhinitis	Cromolyn
Acne	Antiacne tretinoin
	Topical macrolides
Ulcers	Cimetidine
Glaucoma	Ophthalmic miotics
Gout or hyperuricemia	Uric acid agents
High cholesterol	Antilipemics
Migraines	Ergot derivatives
Tuberculosis	Antitubercular agents

Source: Reprinted by permission of the publisher from A Chronic Disease Score from Automated Pharmacy Data, M. Von Korff, E.H. Wagner, and K. Saunders, *Journal of Clinical Epidemiology*, Vol. 45, p. 199. © 1992, Elsevier Science, Inc.

status of prescription drugs to over-the-counter. Inferring diagnoses is also difficult if a disease may be treated with either drugs or other treatments. For example, the measure will not count as high-cholesterol a patient who has been prescribed a low-cholesterol diet rather than drugs. In addition, it does not address some diseases that are often managed on an outpatient basis, such as AIDS.

Ambulatory Care Groups

ACGs use ICD-9 diagnosis codes from administrative insurance claims data to create a case-mix measure to predict utilization of outpatient services. Each ICD-9-CM code is assigned to 1 of 34 ambulatory diagnostic groups (ADGs), which are based on clinical judgments of the stability, chronicity, and expected services use associated with the diagnosis. The ADGs are then further grouped, after intermediate steps, into 51 ACGs, mutually exclusive categories based on number of outpatient visits and total outpatient charges for the period of a year. This measure was validated in a population of adult ambulatory patients (Berlowitz et al., 1995; Weiner et al., 1991).

CONCLUSION

In this chapter, several important issues were emphasized about using comorbidity measures. First, comorbid conditions are diseases other than the principal diagnosis that influence the outcome of treatment. Second, researchers should be wary in adjusting for comorbid diseases, lest they inadvertently adjust for disease or treatment complications and adjust away the outcome of interest. In choosing to use a comorbidity measure rather than a severity of illness measure, the researcher should consider both the study design and the construction of the measure. If the study focuses on one or a few particular diagnoses, a measure of comorbidity will be useful. If the study concerns comparisons of groups but does not focus on specific diseases, the researcher may find a severity of illness measure more appropriate. Finally, an important issue to remember is that measures used to assess comorbidity were often created to assess severity of illness; researchers have adapted these measures as comorbidity measures simply by excluding the disease of primary interest when calculating scores for the measure.

REFERENCES

American Medical Association (1994). *Physician's Current Procedural Terminology*, 4th ed, CPT-4. Chicago: Author.

Berlowitz, D.R., Rosen, A.K., & Moskowitz, M.A. (1995). Ambulatory care casemix measures. *Journal of General Internal Medicine, 10*, 162–170.

Charlson, M.E., Pompei, P., Ales, K.L., & MacKenzie, C.R. (1987). A new method of classifying prognostic comorbidity in longitudinal studies: Development and validation. *Journal of Chronic Diseases, 40*(5), 373–383.

Charlson, M., Szatrowski, T.P., Peterson, J., & Gold, J. (1994). Validation of a combined comorbidity index. *Journal of Clinical Epidemiology, 47*(11), 1,245–1,251.

Clark, D.O., Von Korff, M., Saunders, K., Blauch, W.M., & Simon, G.E. (1995). A chronic disease score with empirically derived weights. *Medical Care, 33*(8), 783–795.

Deyo, R.A., Cherkin D.C., & Ciol, M.A. (1992). Adopting a clinical comorbidity index for use with ICD-9-CM administrative databases. *Journal of Clinical Epidemiology, 45*(6), 613–619.

Greenfield, S., Aronow, H.U., Elashoff, R.M., & Watanabe, D. (1988). Flaws in mortality data: The hazards of ignoring comorbid disease. *JAMA, 260,* 2,253–2,256.

Greenfield, S., Blanco, D.M., Elashoff, R.M., & Ganz, P.A. (1987). Patterns of care related to age of breast cancer patients. *JAMA, 257,* 2,766–2,770.

Greenfield, S., & Nelson, E.C. (1992). Recent developments and future issues in the use of health status assessment measures in clinical settings. *Medical Care, 30*(5), MS23–MS41.

Iezzoni, L. (Ed.). (1994). *Risk adjustment for measuring health outcomes.* Ann Arbor, MI: Health Administration Press.

Iezzoni, L.I., Shwartz, M., Ash, A.S., Mackeiernan, Y., & Hotchkin, E.K. (1994). Risk adjustment methods can affect perceptions of outcomes. *American Journal of Medical Quality, 9*(2), 43–48.

Kahn, K.L., Park, R.E., Brook, R.H., Chassin, M.R., Kosecoff, J., Fink, A., Keesey, J.W., Solomon, D.H. (1988). The effect of comorbidity on appropriateness ratings for two gastrointestinal procedures. *Journal of Clinical Epidemiology, 41*(2), 115–122.

Kaplan, M.H., & Feinstein, A.R. (1974). The importance of classifying initial comorbidity in evaluating the outcome of diabetes mellitus. *Journal of Chronic Disease, 27,* 387–404.

Kennedy, P. (1992). *A Guide to Econometrics, 3rd ed.* Cambridge, MA: The MIT Press, p. 66.

Parkerson, G.R., Broadhead, W.E., & Tse, C.J. (1993). The Duke severity of illness checklist (DUSOI) for measurement of severity and comorbidity. *Journal of Clinical Epidemiology, 46*(4), 379–393.

Romano, P.S., Roos, L.L., & Jollis, J.G. (1993a). Adapting a clinical comorbidity index for use with ICD-9-CM administrative data: Differing perspectives. *Journal of Clinical Epidemiology, 46*(10), 1,075–1,079.

Romano, P.S., Roos, L.L., & Jollis, J.G. (1993b). Further evidence concerning the use of a clinical comorbidity index with ICD-9-CM administrative data. *Journal of Clinical Epidemiology, 46*(10), 1,085–1,090.

Romano, P.S., Roos, L.L., Luft, H.S., Jollis, J.G., Doliszny, K. & the Ischemic Heart Disease Patient Outcomes Research Team. (1994). A comparison of administrative versus clinical data: Coronary artery bypass surgery as an example. *Journal of Clinical Epidemiology, 47*(3), 249–260.

Roos, L.L., Sharp, S.M., & Cohen, M.M. (1991). Comparing clinical information with claims data: Some similarities and differences. *Journal of Clinical Epidemiology, 44*(9), 881–888.

Satariano, W.A. (1992). Comorbidity and functional status in older women with breast cancer: Implications for screening, treatment, and prognosis. *The Journals of Gerontology, 47*(special), 24–31.

Shapiro, M.F, Park, R.E., Keesy, J. & Brook, R.H. (1994). The effect of alternative case-mix adjustments on mortality difference between municipal and voluntary hospitals in New York City. *Health Services Research, 29*(1), 95–112.

U.S. Public Health Service, Health Care Financing Administration. (1980). *The International Classification of Diseases, 9th Revision, Clinical Modification.* PHS 80-1260. Washington, DC: Author.

Verbrugge, L.M., Lepkowski, J.M., & Imanaka, Y. (1989). Comorbidity and its impact on disability. *Milbank Quarterly, 67*(304), 450–484.

Von Korff, M., Wagner, E.H., & Saunders, K.A. (1992). A chronic disease score from automated pharmacy data. *Journal of Clinical Epidemiology, 45,* 197–203.

Weiner, J.P., Starfield, B.H., Steinwachs, D.M., & Mumford, L.M. (1991). Development and application of a population-oriented measure of ambulatory care case-mix. *Medical Care, 29,* 452–472.

NOTES

1. Kennedy (1992, p. 66) explains the importance of considering the sample size and degrees of freedom in a statistical analysis as follows:

   If there are only two observations, a linear function with one independent variable (i.e., two parameters) will fit the data perfectly, *regardless* of what independent variable is used. Adding a third observation will destroy the perfect fit, but the fit will remain quite good, simply because there is effectively only one observation to explain. It is to correct this phenomenon that statistics are adjusted for *degrees of freedom*–the number of "free" or linearly independent observations used in the calculation of the statistic.

2. This measure has subsequently been refined and validated with a sample of 250,000 managed care enrollees (see, Clark, Von Korff, Saunders, Baluch, and Simon, 1995).

8

Demographic and Psychosocial Factors

Stephen Derose

CHAPTER OUTLINE

- What Are Demographic Variables, and Why Are They Measured?
- What Are Psychological and Social Variables, and Why Are They Measured?

The patient or group characteristics relevant to an outcomes study are no different from those used in most clinical studies. Outcomes studies are distinguished by the use of additional measures designed to incorporate a broad perspective on the effects of illness and treatment and account for those factors that may significantly influence treatment and important outcomes. Demographic variables, even more so than psychosocial, have a potential that is often overlooked. Demographic, psychological, and social variables may be risk factors for an illness or other outcome, confounders of results, or modifiers of treatment effect. In addition, some of these variables may even be viewed as outcomes themselves. The *variables of interest* are essentially any characteristics that define the individuals or populations involved in the study and can have an impact on the outcomes. Variables should be included on the basis of an underlying conceptual model that links the variable to the outcomes through a theoretical framework. Some variables, like age and sex, seem to be regularly addressed as if by force of tradition. Taking these variables for granted may lead to loss of important information that might have been obtained with more thoughtful application and adherence to a well-developed conceptual model. Unlike severity of illness and comorbidity measures, the information contained in demographic, psychological, and social variables exists in every individual, independently of the presence of illness.

175

When choosing among the many demographic and psychosocial variables to measure, investigators must consider not only their own goals but the interests and demands of a broader audience, which may include health care providers and health plan managers and policy makers. In some cases, it may be important to show that a given variable, such as sex or race, is not significantly related to the outcomes. An approach that restricts the number of variables selected to those considered of proven importance runs the risk of criticism of results because of unmeasured factors postulated as significant. This consideration is particularly relevant in research areas that are not already well developed. An approach that attempts to measure everything possible, however, can be inefficient, costly, and clouded by areas of poor data of uncertain significance. The selection of which variables to measure in a particular study will depend on a balance between practical considerations and a cautious assessment of what information is needed to evaluate convincingly the hypothesis under question within its theoretical framework. The following discussion is intended to expand the reader's understanding of common demographic and psychosocial variables so that they may be meaningfully applied in a conceptual model capable of driving outcomes research.

The variables chosen will define the study population for the purpose of drawing conclusions from the results. When a randomized study design is not possible, establishing relevant baseline characteristics of study groups aids in validating an argument that study results are due to the differences in interventions between groups and not to confounding factors that are distributed unequally between groups. Describing a study population's baseline characteristics also allows researchers to generalize results to similar patient populations. Looking at the contribution of individual variables through statistical methods may identify key factors in determining the outcome of interest. Analysis based on these variables may define patient subgroups in which the intervention is more or less effective or uncover an important interaction between risk factors. This can be used to predict outcomes, to aid in determining treatment strategies for different populations, and to inform the choice between treatment options at the individual patient care level.

WHAT ARE DEMOGRAPHIC VARIABLES, AND WHY ARE THEY MEASURED?

Demographic variables traditionally are viewed as characteristics that define a population in terms of its size, the elements that compose it, and its geographic distribution. Demographic variables may be seen as more concrete, distinct states in comparison to psychosocial variables, which represent a highly individualized and subjective measurement of a concept, such as social support, often along a spectrum. Individuals may be described in part by demographic characteristics and study groups described in part by the summation of the characteristics of the individual subjects. Traditional epidemiological variables include age, sex, ethnic group, race, socioeconomic status, occupation, and marital status.

These variables are used in several ways. They can define the study population to generalize from results and to demonstrate to the greatest extent possible the validity of the results. This latter purpose is achieved by controlling for these factors during analysis to isolate the intervention effect. Outcomes studies may use these variables to determine which patient characteristics are associated with better or worse outcomes, analogous to risk factor determinations in epidemiological studies of disease causation. Additional uses stemming from observational studies may include predicting resource consumption when interventions are planned for a new population or adjusting reimbursement for services based on the characteristics of populations served by an intervention. Some demographic variables may even be at least secondary outcomes of interest, such as changes in marital status or employment status that occur with illness.

Variables are often chosen because they have a logical or historical association to the outcomes of interest or because they are easy to measure. Some variables, such as sex and age, are nearly always measured because they have a history of significance across many different types of illness and interventions. Historical precedent, however, should not deter the investigator from considering the contribution of these and similar demographic variables in the theoretical framework. Some variables will be surrogates for one or more unmeasured factors of interest. For example, age can be a surrogate for comorbidity, sex for social roles, and socioeconomic status may represent an aggregate of many other variables, such as lifestyle factors, stress levels, access to care, and so forth. These aggregated or summary variables are still useful in assessing risk and adjusting for confounding, but greater caution must be used in interpreting their relation to study results. Even when there is a strong association of an aggregate variable, such as socioeconomic status to an outcome of interest, assumptions about *causal* association must be made very cautiously since the association may be driven by only one of several variables that contribute to the aggregate measure.

How Might Demographic Variables Be Classified?

Assignment of variables to categories can make the possible mechanisms of effect and the interrelationship of different variables more apparent. Classification of demographic variables into mutually exclusive, neat categories, however, is problematic. Variables that can be viewed as aggregated sets of many factors may defy easy classification into even the simplest of schemes. Some suggestions for organizing thinking about variables of interest follow.

A commonly used epidemiological classification scheme divides variables into host versus environmental factors (Mausner & Kramer, 1985). *Host factors*, such as genetic makeup, affect susceptibility to illness and response to interventions and may include necessary and/or sufficient causes of illness. Environmental factors, such as culturally specific dietary practices, affect exposure to causal and modifying factors for illness and response to interventions. A demographic classification scheme uses the categories of *biosocial* (where traits are viewed as ascribed) and *sociocultural* (where traits are primarily achieved and characterize an individual's position in society; Pol & Thomas, 1992). Similarly, variables could be described and categorized as *determined* or *acquired*. *Determined variables* are not amenable to change or choice and represent facts present out of biological necessity. In this category are age, sex, birth cohort, race, and ethnicity (genetic heritage component). *Acquired variables* are theoretically amenable to change or choice and do not result from biological necessity, although genetic factors may play a role. Included are socioeconomic status, education and literacy, occupation and employment status, marital status, religion, place of residence, and the cultural or religious components of ethnicity. Some details of measurement are provided with the discussions of the variables.

Which Demographic Variables Are Measured?

Age

Age is an important variable to consider, and it is relatively easy to collect. The National Center for Health Statistics maintains data for U.S. mortality and morbidity by age. There is an increasing prevalence of most chronic diseases with aging, and the incidence of many acute conditions, such as injuries, decreases with age. Because age is also accompanied by declines in functional status and recuperative skills (Pol & Thomas, 1992), outcomes may be expected to be worse in older age groups. Also, complications of care are often greater in older adults (Iezzoni, 1994). Longer hospital stays and more complications can lead to increased costs of care. These effects make the age distribution important for many studies.

Age can often be an *independent risk factor*, meaning that an association with an outcome persists even after statistical adjustment for all other known risk factors, such as comorbid conditions. This is evident in the use of age as a variable in the Acute Physiology and Chronic Health Evaluation (APACHE III) and similar measures (Iezzoni, 1994). Of course, age as an unadjusted variable can represent other factors that may affect outcome, such as functional status, socioeconomic status, employment, and compliance.

Age can be interpreted in various ways: one could conceptualize age as not just chronological but as a physiologic or functional age, depending on the conceptual model employed. An investigator may be primarily interested in the division of subjects by the standard retirement age of 65 rather than specific birth dates. It is easily collected as a continuous variable, and it is usually better to collect the data in this form even if a categorical analysis is envisioned.

It should also be remembered that when looking at the effects of age on an outcome or adjusting for age between study groups, the methods used in data analysis can affect the relationships seen. For example, when using age as a categorical variable, the choice of age range used in analysis can determine how strong a relationship is observed between age and the outcome, which may further affect choices about adjusting for age in the analysis. The possibility of an age bias should be considered in reviewing studies or planning a new trial, since the age of a patient may affect the treatment type or intensity offered to a patient.

Sex

Sex is another important characteristic to record and analyze. In general, women have been noted to have higher levels of morbidity and men higher levels of mortality, for both acute and chronic conditions. When various social factors are controlled, the morbidity differential appears to lessen, whereas the mortality differential remains (Verbrugge, 1989). Population data for disease distribution by sex in the United States are available from the National Center for Health Statistics. Women tend to be more frequent users of health services (Cockerham, 1986). The importance of sex will often be disease specific. The differences seen between men and women may be due to different habits in seeking care, the sex-specific natural course of the disease, or social role factors. Gender differences in diagnosis and reporting have been especially prominent in the mental health arena, where the debate over "nature versus nurture" has been intense: rates of neurosis and manic-depression are consistently higher for women, and rates of personality disorders are consistently higher in men (Dohrenwend & Dohrenwend, 1976). It is generally not known if the differences seen in mental health diagnoses, as well as other conditions, reflect primarily anatomic and physiologic differences between men and women or the effects of socialization and societal roles. Verbrugge (1989) provides a brief review of the notable sex differences in mental health and the psychosocial factors that contribute to these observations. Due to important historical lifestyle differences between men and women, the sex variable may be incorporating the effects of unmeasured social or lifestyle factors that can confound the relationship between sex and outcome, such as higher rates of alcohol use and smoking in men.

Sex differences, while clearly important in long-term risks due to differences in disease prevalence, are often not powerful predictors for short-term outcomes. For example, sex does not predict survival in intensive care unit (ICU) patients in the well-established APACHE III measure (Iezzoni, 1994). Sex can affect access to care, in terms of both seeking help and receiving it. When examining sex effects in a nonrandomized study design, careful attention must be given to the possibility of selection bias. Even if bias is not evident in the primary treatment, it may be wise to consider the possibility that different secondary or ancillary treatments were given based on the sex of the patient. Studies today are being more carefully designed to include adequate numbers of both men and women to look for sex-based differences in outcomes.

As a final note, gender and sex are not interchangeable terms among the research community. *Sex* corresponds to physical anatomy and the typical physiological differences between men and women. Depending on the research needs, sex may be specified at a chromosomal level, with the presence of XX versus XY, although other combinations, such as genetic mosaics, may lead to unexpected difficulty in definition. *Gender* is often used to mean sex or gender role identification, especially in sociological or psychological research. For instance, psychological tests may reveal some (normal) men and women who identify more closely with the normative response set of the opposite sex. This would be considered evidence of mixed or opposite gender identification and, in fact, may be more predictive of behaviors than the more simple identification of an individual as male or female from a survey question. The carefully conceived conceptual model will determine the use of the sex or gender variable in the outcomes study.

Race and Ethnicity

Race and ethnicity as predictive variables are closely related, but there are important distinctions. Each contains components from both biologic and social spheres. Traditionally, *race* is meant to refer to a group of people who share a set of physical characteristics and who presumably share an ancestral heritage from a particular region of the world. In practice, the identification of race is nebulous due to the heterogeneity of members (e.g., Asians or Europeans) and the intermingling of races in many modern societies. *Ethnicity* refers to a common cultural heritage. Certain ethnic groups may have a shared genetic makeup due to ancestral heritage from a particular geographic region or to reproductive isolation. The importance of race and ethnicity as variables probably has much more to do with the socioeconomic correlates of that status in a particular society rather than genetic factors. Independence of race and ethnicity from other risk factors for illness is rarely clear due to the close association with socioeconomic status, education, employment, and lifestyle habits. In fact, part of what may determine an ethnic group are lifestyle habits.

The variables of race and ethnicity can be used in an epidemiological way to identify groups in society that are at greater risk of disease or adverse outcome. This serves the purpose of improving public health by identifying areas of need. In outcomes studies or other clinical research, we may use these variables in a similar way to find subgroups who respond to treatment differently or are at higher risk for adverse outcomes. Additionally, we can look at the contribution of these and other variables in determining the observed outcome to see the effect of race or ethnicity after correction for other measured variables. Correcting observed associations between race, ethnicity, and outcome for other factors, such as socioeconomic status or dietary practices, serves to isolate the residual, independent effect of race or ethnicity and addresses the mechanisms behind the observed associations. This could be viewed as an attempt to focus on the genetic components of these variables, which improves our understanding of the mechanisms of illness and its treatment. Certain diseases are linked to genetic status as either a unique cause of disease, such as the gene for a hemoglobin variant in sickle-cell anemia, or as a contributing factor and part of a "web of causation" for disease, such as certain lipid abnormalities and atherosclerotic vascular disease. Sometimes race or ethnicity may be tapping this genetically determined, biologic contribution to an illness. To determine the genetic factors involved in an illness or treatment, however, specific genetic studies need to be performed.

Racial differences in general health measures in U.S. society are pronounced, particularly between Americans of African and European descent. When compared to white Americans, black Americans have higher rates of morbidity for essentially every major disease, as well as increased overall mortality and decreased life expectancy. Through 1988, ischemic heart disease was the only major cause of morbidity and mortality where white male mortality rates exceeded black male mortality rates. Since that time, improvements in mortality rates were seen for both races, but the rate in whites lowered to a greater extent than the rate in blacks. This caused a shift in relative order to the point where the mortality rate in black males now exceeds that in white males for this *International Classification of Diseases* (ICD) (U.S. Public Health Service, 1980) code as well (National Center for Health Statistics, morbidity and mortality data). Higher levels of disability by various measures are also reported among blacks in the United States (Pol & Thomas, 1992). Socioeconomic status has a large impact on the observed differences in black and white mortality levels (Navarro, 1991).

The United States is the only major Western industrialized nation that does not routinely collect information on income, education, or occupation with mortality statistics. Where this has been done, the differences in mortality between high and low socioeconomic status are far greater than the differences seen between the different races occupying the same social class (Navarro, 1991). The fact that socioeconomic status likely confounds the relationship between race and health indicators does not affect the usefulness of this demographic variable in identifying higher risk populations. Generally speaking, Asians have morbidity and mortality rates between those of white and black Americans (Pol & Thomas, 1992). Native Americans are at high risk of morbidity and mortality for many conditions, such as diabetes and tuberculosis. Hispanics show a mixed risk profile compared to the general white population (Cockerham, 1986). A standard, modern categorization scheme for recording race is used in the U.S. Public Health Service grant application, shown in Table 8–1. Descriptions of the categorization scheme to minimize misunderstanding and inaccurate or missing data are recommended. Again, selection bias for diagnosis and treatment must be considered in reviewing and conducting research related to racial or ethnic status.

Socioeconomic Status

Socioeconomic status is a concept that can be difficult to operationalize. Unlike the variables of age, sex, and race, an individual's socioeconomic status can be determined in some part by his or her behavior (Dohrenwend, 1990). It reflects positions in society that differ in education, income, occupation, area of residence, and issues of lifestyle. These factors indicate the amount of power and resources available to a person (Mausner & Kramer, 1985).

Table 8–1 Race and Ethnic Classification

Race and/or Ethnic Origin	Description
American Indian or Alaskan Native	A person having origins in any of the original peoples of North America and who maintains a cultural identification through tribal affiliation or community recognition
Asian or Pacific Islander	A person having origins in any of the original peoples of the Far East, Southeast Asia, the Indian subcontinent, or the Pacific Islands
Black, not of Hispanic origin	A person having origins in any of the black racial groups of Africa
Hispanic	A person of Mexican, Puerto Rican, Cuban, Central or South American, or other Spanish culture or origin, regardless of race
White, not of Hispanic origin	A person having origins in any of the original peoples of Europe, North Africa, or the Middle East

Note: The category that most closely reflects the individual's recognition in the community should be used when reporting mixed racial and/or ethnic origins.
Source: Reprinted from U.S. Public Health Service Grant Application (PHS 398), United States Health Resources and Services Administration.

Socioeconomic status can be a powerful predictor in outcomes studies. The most commonly used indicators of status are income, occupation, and education. Measurement is made problematic by the fact that an individual may change socioeconomic status or be categorized as higher status by some measures and lower status by others, such as high education and low income (Pol & Thomas, 1992). Not directly measured by these indicators, but closely correlated to socioeconomic status, are extremely important lifestyle factors, such as diet, habits such as smoking, perceptions and attitudes, access to care, and exposure to environmental (including social) hazards. If investigators are specifically interested in any of these factors, they should be directly measured. Social scientists generally divide society into at least three levels: lower, middle, and upper. In Britain, six levels of social class have been defined and used by the government: professional; intermediate; nonmanual, skilled; manual, skilled; partly skilled; and unskilled (Mausner & Kramer, 1985). The conceptual model guiding the outcomes study should be developed to include explicit reasons for measuring socioeconomic status by the specific indicators chosen.

Income seems at first glance to be a relatively easily applied indicator of socioeconomic status, but even this measure is not straightforward. *The Methods and Materials of Demography* provides information about the subtle issues in obtaining an accurate measurement of this and several other demographic variables (Shryock et al., 1976). For example, income can be measured as personal or family. An estimate of gross income is the goal, and this ideally includes all regular yearly earnings but not one-time gains. Household incomes are considered to be measured best by combining the incomes of individuals rather than asking about the total. The socioeconomic status of nonworking household members such as children and homemakers is best indicated by the family variable. Some developing countries or very poor people may rely heavily on noncash sources of income. Additionally, some people may be unwilling to respond or will give misleading answers to such a personal question. Supplying a categorical response set, rather than using a continuous format where the respondent is asked to specify an income, may improve compliance. Family income measures may be improved by using the federal government's poverty index, which adjusts for family size and cost of living (Liberatos, Link, & Kelsey, 1988). The 1985 to 1989 U.S. National Health Interview Survey (NHIS) used the income categorization scheme shown in Exhibit 8–1 (U.S. Public Health Service, 1987).

In general, decreasing incomes are associated with increasing prevalence of acute and chronic conditions and worsening measures of health status and outcomes, including self-reported health. The severity of conditions is likely to be greater in lower income groups. Increased disability has been assessed by various measures, such as work-loss days (Pol & Thomas, 1992). Increased hospitalization rates in the poor for potentially avoidable conditions have been demonstrated (Weissman, Gastsonis, & Epstein, 1992). There have been examples of longer

Exhibit 8–1 Income Categories Using 1985–1989 U.S. NHIS

Income	
Less than $1,000 (including loss)	$25,000–$29,999
$1,000–$1,999	$30,000–$34,999
$2,000–$2,999	$35,000–$39,999
(increasing by $1,000 increments	$40,000–$44,999
to $19,999)	$45,000–$49,999
$20,000–$24,999	$50,000 and over

hospital stays and less intensive care for patients of lower socioeconomic status with specific medical conditions (Epstein et al., 1988). In the mental health arena, older as well as more recent research has demonstrated an inverse association of socioeconomic status with schizophrenia, antisocial personality, and substance abuse (Dohrenwend, 1990). Suicide is more common in the higher social classes (Pol & Thomas, 1992). The associations seen between socioeconomic status and mental health may be explained by social conditions causing disease, social drift of the diseased person into lower status, or a combination of both.

Education, as another indicator of socioeconomic status, shows a similar pattern to income in its association with illness and health measures. The usual method is to measure the highest level of education achieved. This may be defined in different ways: by type of institution (grade school, high school, college, graduate school), by the number of years of education, the highest grade achieved, or the age at completion of full-time education (Abramson, 1990). The increasing prevalence of higher educational attainment over the past few generations in U.S. society makes comparisons over widely different age groups problematic. A definition that most practically and best suits the purposes of the research should be sought. Literacy may also be used as a basic measure of education. It is defined by the United Nations as the ability of a person both to read and to write, with understanding, a short, simple statement on his or her everyday life. The data on literacy are acquired by verbally asking a person if he or she can read and write. In a country with high levels of literacy, many illiterate people may be hesitant to answer this question accurately (Shryock et al., 1976).

Occupation, in addition to its role as a leading indicator of socioeconomic status (as in the British social class definitions), may demonstrate a unique pattern of association with disease. This is observed because of the exposure of certain professions to disease risks and the propensity of certain person-types to specific occupations. For example, miners have exposure to dust and fumes that can cause several types of lung disease. A study of London public transportation employees demonstrated that sedentary workers (the drivers) had a higher risk of fatal coronary events than those working at a job that required higher levels of physical activity (the conductors; Morris & Heady, 1953a, 1953b). High-risk jobs, such as mining and construction work, may attract personality types that are risk taking, just as physically undemanding jobs may attract sedentary workers or those whose health is poor. It may be difficult to tell the contribution of personal factors versus environmental in the association of occupation type and disease, such as the high rates of suicide seen among psychiatrists (Pol & Thomas, 1992). Occupations of lower status and prestige are characterized by the same trends seen in the poor and uneducated (Pol & Thomas, 1992). Occupation may be defined as present or usual occupation, training, or actual work performed. For those retired or unemployed, that status or past primary occupation may be measured, depending on which seems most relevant (Abramson, 1990).

The status of unemployment is a significant risk factor for the increased morbidity and mortality seen among the poor. The unemployed include persons who, at the time of the study period, were seeking work. It also includes persons temporarily not seeking work because of illness or future work arrangements. To be categorized as employed or unemployed, a person must be economically active. The noneconomically active include students, homemakers, and recipients of incomes from other sources, such as property (Shryock et al., 1976). Although it is often unclear if illness leads to unemployment and poverty, or vice versa, the association is still useful in identifying high-risk groups and making risk adjustments in analyses of results.

Composite measures of socioeconomic status exist that attempt to combine occupation, education, and income into a single score. One advantage of using a composite index is to improve comparability between studies. Duncan's Socioeconomic Index is the most frequently used measure. It is based primarily on public opinion about occupational prestige from a national survey (Liberatos et al., 1988). Hollingshead's Index of Social Position is another composite measure with a history of widespread use, and it is based on occupational rank and educational attainment (Liberatos et al., 1988).

Marital Status

Marital status, unlike age, sex, and socioeconomic status, is not frequently considered as a risk factor in models of illness, although marital status has been linked to heath status and health-related behaviors. Married people tend to score better on general indicators of mental and physical health and have lower morbidity and mortality than other marital status groups (Pol & Thomas, 1992). The distinction in health status appears to be primarily between married versus not married (Burman & Margolin, 1992), although, in 1979, a study based on health surveys and census data found that divorced and separated people had the worst health status, followed by widowed then single individuals, with married people being the healthiest (Verbrugge, 1979). With cardiovascular disease, for example, a study in the Netherlands demonstrated a relative risk of total and coronary mortality significantly higher in never-married men than in those who were married (Mendes de Leon et al., 1992). Additionally, once ill, marital status seems to affect health outcomes positively. Ten-year survival among white women with breast cancer was better in those who were married at presentation for therapy than in those who were widowed, after adjustment for age, socioeconomic status, stage of disease, and delay in seeking treatment (Neale, Tilley, & Vernon, 1986). Married men and women hospitalized for acute myocardial infarction had significantly decreased hospital fatality rates and 10-year mortality compared to those unmarried at the time of hospitalization, with adjustment for other factors (Chandra et al., 1983). Self-reported disability days are fewer for married people than for other groups in the NHIS (U.S. Public Health Service, 1987). The transition from married to divorced or widowed is associated with increases in morbidity and mortality (Pol & Thomas, 1992).

A person's status is generally characterized as never married, married, divorced, or widowed. The United Nations classification is: single and never married, married and not legally separated, widowed and not remarried, divorced and not remarried, and married but legally separated. Couples living together are often counted as married, while separated married couples are treated variably. In addition to marital status, some work has been done with marital quality, which represents a subjective evaluation of the marital relationship, and marital interaction, which generally represents objective assessment of marital behavior (Burman & Margolin, 1992). It should be remembered that those who are unhealthy may tend to be single, selecting out a healthier, married group. Marital status may change with the onset of health problems, although there is little research data at present to support this supposition (Burman & Margolin, 1992). A successful marriage usually provides a strong degree of social support and stress buffering. The marital status variable may represent this as well as lifestyle factors, such as dietary practices or smoking, different rates and time frames in seeking care for illness, insurance coverage, or a host of other factors. Whatever the reasons for the associations observed, the summary nature of this and other variables does not affect predictive ability or much of the usefulness in risk factor adjustment. When studying the etiology of illness, however, we may not know the specific factors involved in that measure that are ultimately responsible for the association seen. This limitation should not detract from developing a theoretical framework that includes a specific measurement of the variable because it is only in this way that its information potential is maximized.

Religion

Religion as a variable associated with disease and outcomes is not as well studied as the preceding variables, although a large body of literature exists going back over a long period of time. Probably the most clear association of religious affiliation and illness has been demonstrated by observational studies. For example, Seventh Day Adventists in California have lower coronary heart disease rates than other Californians, although the effect of traditional risk factors remains qualitatively similar among the Adventists (Fraser et al., 1992). Utah Mormons have lower rates for all causes of cancer compared to non-Mormons in Utah and the general U.S. population (Lyon, Gardner, & Gress, 1994). These effects may be attributable to differences in health-related practices, such as diet and smoking. Patient treatment choices may be affected by religion, as in the decision to have an abortion, or the avoidance of blood products by Jehovah's Witnesses.

Outcomes may also be influenced by religion. A recent study demonstrated less maternal complications and neonatal intensive care unit admissions in patients belonging to two Christian groupings than in those with no religious affiliation. This relationship existed after correction for a number of (but not all potentially significant) confounding factors, which is often the case in these studies (King, Hueston, & Rudy, 1994). A review by Levin (1994) found substantial evidence for an association of religion and health across many types of studies in different regions and time periods. There appears to be lower risk of morbidity and mortality, and trends toward better health status indicators for many common diseases in the more behaviorally strict religions or denominations and in individuals with higher levels of religious involvement. Whether this association is causal, rather than a result of confounders, is still very much in question (Levin, 1994). The positive association of religious attendance with better health as demonstrated by several studies can be questioned on the basis of good health leading to more frequent attendance. (Levin & Vanderpool, 1987). The religious dimension could be, and has been, considered a part of treatment. A double-blind clinical trial of intercessory prayer showed a (borderline) nonsignificant but positive effect of prayer on improving the outcomes of two chronic diseases (Joyce, Welldon, & Litt, 1965).

Religion may be defined as religious or spiritual belief preference, whether or not there is a recognized, organized group, or as affiliation with an established group that has specified tenets (Shryock et al., 1976). Both religious preference, as defined above, and practice habits may be important. *Religiosity* may be considered the degree of religious commitment in terms of attitudes and practices. Some common measures of religiosity are frequency of religious attendance, church membership, and subjective self-ratings of religiosity (Levin, 1994). Even the measure of religious attendance is far from straightforward—different religious traditions will have different frequencies of attendance of social gatherings, and other meetings, such as classes and small gatherings at home, could be important in certain traditions (Levin & Vanderpool, 1987). Additionally, the past use of the frequency variable itself has been on a scale that is heavily skewed toward one extreme. Religious service attendance has often been measured as weekly or more, two to three times per month, and less often. Around 40% of the U.S. population attends religious services at least weekly, making the distribution of responses for most populations non-normal and leading to significant problems with standard statistical analysis (Levin & Vanderpool, 1987). Levin and Vanderpool provide a revised scale of frequency of religious attendance and, most importantly, a theoretical framework for the variable of religion. To measure fully and carefully the complex religion variable, it is advised to measure attendance to other meetings and functions; particular religious affiliation, including denomination or body; geographical location and duration of residence; current age; age at significant rites of passage; self-rated religious commitment; and a religiosity scale appropriate to the specific religious traditions of the study subjects (Levin & Vanderpool, 1987).

Religion may represent the effect of ethnic and lifestyle habits (such as genetic heritage, diet, sexual, and other norms), psychological and social support (through faith, belief systems, participation in rites and community practices), or other factors. Considering the degree of religious belief in the United States, with Gallup polls demonstrating that 95% of the general public believes in God, there has been a dearth of research in this area in mental health and medicine in general (Sherrill & Larson, 1988). With a history of organized religious persecution within the lifetime of many persons of certain faiths, such as Judaism, investigators should realize that there may be some hesitation among individuals to respond to religious orientation questions in a survey or census.

Other Variables

Some additional variables are worth consideration, depending on the study. Place of origin by country and region may give information similar to ethnicity but possibly other information as well, such as a history of exposures to agents common to a region. Years of residence in the current region or history of immigration and migration may be relevant in studies on exposure to risk factors or interventions or simply as measures of stability. Urban versus rural residency affects access to physicians (e.g., low numbers of obstetricians in rural America) and some high-technology services. Language, defined as that with which a person was raised or primarily speaks, may indicate ethnic or regional origin or affect ability to follow treatment directions. Variables such as maternal age and parity, one- or two-parent family, family size and crowding index, birth order, and others may be necessary in studies of natality or child health. Along with the more essential variables noted above, any demographic variable is justified if the researcher has a reasonable expectation of predictive ability on the outcome of interest, if it is necessary to characterize the groups for purposes of comparison or generalization of results, and if there exists a reasonable means of measurement. All these variables should be placed in the context of the conceptual model that drives the outcomes study.

WHAT ARE PSYCHOLOGICAL AND SOCIAL VARIABLES, AND WHY ARE THEY MEASURED?

Historically, improvements in the overall health of society due to scientific advances appear to be slowing, particularly for basic measures, such as mortality rates and life span. This may be due less to the efficacy of health care interventions than to the inability to change the fundamental behaviors of people or the inertia of the socioeconomic and political environment. The psychological and social variables measured in outcomes studies are indicators of concepts that influence psychosocial well-being and patient behavior. *Psychosocial variables* are psychological, social, and interrelated factors that pertain to the individual and must be measured using some form of developed indicators (e.g., a scale). These variables encompass a broad range of patient characteristics that include comprehension of the illness state and interventions; mental well-being; ability and willingness to comply with treatment and to interact with providers of care; social health; and support networks.

Variables of mental health, social health, and psychological well-being are important factors in acquiring illness, seeking treatment, and responding to care. Their importance will vary depending on the individual and the type of illness. For example, mildly depressed mood in a person taking antibiotics for a bladder infection would not be expected to affect care as much as clinically diagnosed depression in a diabetic patient who needs to monitor and treat him- or herself on a continual basis to avoid serious adverse health effects. Measuring these variables helps researchers estimate their significance in determining health outcomes and allows for adjustment of the effects of other variables of interest. In addition, psychological and social variables can be just as much an outcome of interest as a risk factor for illness. With other measures of health status, they can reveal important things about the effects of an intervention. Depression provides a good example of a condition that can affect the outcomes of therapy and be an independent outcome of interest—this might occur in drug therapy utilizing beta blockers, with their tendency for the side effect of depression.

How Might Psychological and Social Variables Be Measured and Characterized?

Measurement of psychological and social health can be difficult to put into practice or operationalize. A variable exists on two levels: the concept you wish to measure, which is part of the theoretical construct that motivates the research, and the operationalization of this concept through one or several measurable factors that represent the concept of interest. These operationalized variables will be associated with sets of data gathered from the study, and they will be used in the statistical analysis. Data can come from several sources: self-reports (includes subjective feelings or self-monitoring), reports from significant others (their feelings, observations, or ratings), or reports from a trained professional (ratings, observations, or more open-ended assessments). Some measures aim at discrimination of qualitatively different states, such as major depressive illness versus depressed feelings, while others quantitatively rate respondents along a continuum with no referral to a concept of qualitative differences. Evidence of good reliability and validity in a measure increases the likelihood that conclusions based on its application will be valid. Validity and reliability have very specific meaning in relation to the measurement of an abstract concept through a scale. (A discussion of these and related measurement issues can be found in Chapter 9.)

Choosing the best measurement scale for the psychosocial variables of interest is an important skill. Scales are often created to meet the specific needs of a study, but, over time, a growing body of well-conceived scales has been developed and widely applied. These commonly used scales are the best place to start when a specific measurement is desired. Using widely applied scales may promote easier comparisons between studies, making results more easily grasped by the diverse audience reading medical outcomes studies. When an appropriate measurement tool does not exist, then a scale can be developed or modified as necessary. Whenever a scale is modified significantly or applied in a new setting, an argument for its applicability is necessary, and the reliability and validity in that setting must be reconsidered.

Health sciences research has yielded many variations of measures and uniquely developed scales for specific studies; there are literally several hundreds of health behavior and psychosocial measurement scales in the literature. Choosing a scale without the aid of a local expert in the area of interest can be a daunting task. The following section reviews salient features of several scales from the areas of mental health, social health, and general psychological well-being. It is not intended as a comprehensive reference but, rather, as a starting place to become familiar with features of common and useful scales and to help the reader understand some of the depth, breadth, and types of scales available in a particular area. For more information on the development, purpose, and details of applying the following measures, readers should refer to the original references. For a review of the pertinent literature and assessment of the evidence for use of a measure in a particular population or setting and a detailed summary of evidence for reliability and validity, readers are referred to texts such as those by McDowell and Wilkin (McDowell & Newell, 1996; Wilkin, Hallem, & Doggett, 1992).

Psychosocial variables can be categorized into the following domains:

- psychological morbidity and health (concerned with mental illness, health, and general psychological well-being)
- social health
- various health beliefs, attitudes, or behaviors

The way these variables are measured is reflective of the underlying theory that explains their influence on health. An investigator's choice of variable and measurement technique is determined by the conceptual model, which specifies the relationships between potentially influential factors and the outcomes of interest. The scales chosen for review here are devoted to the measurement of a single concept and are, therefore, *unidimensional* in nature. Measures of general health often include a few items from the domains of psychosocial variables. (These broad measures are detailed in Chapter 2, "Generic Measures.")

Which Psychological and Social Variables Are Measured?

Measures of psychological morbidity and health extend along a spectrum from states of illness to states of wellness. The goal is to determine some measurable characteristic indicative of mental or psychological health and illness. The following discussion focuses primarily on the spectrum of emotional/psychological function below the level of formal diagnosis of mental disorder (the range of psychological morbidity from screening for detection of a diseased state to identification of a normal state of health). This focus will envelop the needs of most outcomes studies. A diagnosed mental disorder such as an anxiety syndrome is considered a qualitatively different state from the spectrum of anxious mood changes that a normal individual might experience. Studies of mental illness will need severity measures specifically designed for that illness. (For a general discussion, see Chapter 6, "Severity.") Covered here are the well-established variables of depression, anxiety, and general well-being. Many of these measures incorporate components that are factors in the measurement of a closely related variable, such as questions about feelings of both stress and anxiety in depression scales. This overlap occurs because symptoms may coexist across different conditions in many subjects. This observation serves to demonstrate another point about quantifying or categorizing concepts. Measures developed empirically, based on symptoms observed or self-reported in patients, may be measuring several distinct conditions that vary from the norms of human behavior and are, therefore, more likely to be tapping different underlying concepts or constructs (McDowell & Newell, 1996). This overlap can result in scales sensitive to aberration from the norm but not very specific in measuring the intended variable. A scale that originates from a theoretical construct and represents it well will have the potential for greater validity and specificity, assuming the construct is truly applicable to the problem.

Depression Scales

Depression is a well-studied entity with a diverse group of measures. Different forms of depression exist, from mild mood swings to persistent major depression with physical ramifications. The goal of the research and the study population dictate the appropriate choice of scale. The measure chosen must be sensitive to changes in depression in the population to which it is applied. People of lower socioeconomic status, for example, are believed to express depression more through physical complaints, whereas those of higher socioeconomic status tend to express affective complaints (McDowell & Newell, 1996). Depression in older adults may manifest differently than in the young or pediatric populations, so different measures may be needed. Some measures are considered better for screening purposes, with a high sensitivity to depression, whereas others were designed to identify and characterize the severity of major depression or a change in clinical status. Scales used formally to diagnose depression are not covered here—the emphasis is on the range of depressive symptoms. Psychological (e.g., hopelessness, loss of pleasure), somatic (e.g., sleep disorder, loss of appetite), or behavioral (e.g., withdrawal from social activities, work performance) dimensions may be queried. As is evident in the following discussion, sometimes the predominant use of a scale over time does not always correspond to the original intent of that measure. Several examples of established scales follow, and Table 8–2 summarizes the major attributes of these commonly used depression measures.

The Beck Depression Inventory. Designed to measure the behavioral manifestations of depression, the Beck Depression Inventory (BDI) follows from clinical observations and measures many features of depression considered important in the *Diagnostic and Statistical Manual of the American Psychological Association* (Beck et al., 1961). There are 21 items, and it can be used in an interview or can be self-administered in 5 to 10 minutes. Revisions exist, and a short form was developed as a rapid screening tool (Beck & Beck, 1972). Reliability and validity are both considered generally good in the various settings tested (McDowell & Newell, 1996). Foreign language translations exist. Guidelines for cut-points for defining depression may be varied depending on the population and setting in order to balance sensitivity with concerns about false positives (McDowell & Newell, 1996). Commentators have had concerns about low specificity, and clinical diagnoses of depression should be based on further evaluation. It is considered a sensitive tool, however, and appropriate for depression screening.

Table 8–2 Overview of Selected Depression Scales

Measurement Scale	Intent*	Population†	Setting‡	Uses§	Administration	Items/Time
Beck Depression Inventory (Beck et al., 1961)	Degree of behavioral manifestations	Psychiatric, general	Inpatient, outpatient	Screening	Self, interviewer	21/5–10 Min.
Center for Epidemiologic Studies Depression Scale (Radloff, 1977)	Detection in general population	General, psychiatric, other patients	Community, outpatient	Screening	Self	20/10–15 Min.
Geriatric Depression Scale (Yesavage & Brink, 1983)	Detection in older adults	Older adults	Community, clinic, institutional	Screening	Self	30/8–10 Min.
Hamilton Rating Scale for Depression (Hamilton, 1960, 1967)	Severity in previously diagnosed patients	Depressed patients	Various clinical	Severity assessment, change monitoring	Clinician, other interviewer	21/30+ Min.
Montgomery-Åsberg Depression Rating Scale (Montgomery & Åsberg, 1979)	Detection of treatment effect	Depressed patients	Inpatient and outpatient	Change, severity monitoring	Clinician	10/20–60 Min.

*Original intention of the authors in developing their measure of depression.
†Population for which the measure was developed and the general population types in which the measure has been subsequently applied.
‡Environment in which the measure was originally applied or general environments in which the measure has been subsequently applied.
§Types of applications for which the measure was developed or later used. Often the primary use that has developed over time does not correspond to the original intent.

The Center for Epidemiologic Studies Depression Scale. Created to measure the affective components of depression, the Center for Epidemiologic Studies Depression Scale (CES-D) was designed to detect depression in the general population (Radloff, 1977). There are 20 items, and it is self-administered, taking from 10 to 15 minutes to complete. A short form is available (Andresen et al., 1994). Reliability is good, although retest reliability can be low; validity is considered good (McDowell & Newell, 1996). Foreign language translations exist. Population standards have been estimated for a broad range of ages and for different demographic characteristics (McDowell & Newell, 1996). As with the BDI, there are concerns about low specificity and a high false-positive rate, although sensitivity appears to be good, making this a good screening instrument for the general population. Formal diagnoses of depression would require confirmatory interviews.

The Geriatric Depression Scale. Designed primarily as a screening test for depression in older adults, the Geriatric Depression Scale focuses on affective symptoms rather than the potentially less reliable psychomotor and cognitive symptoms, which can be confused with normal aging and illness (Yesavage & Brink, 1983). The scale was intended for clinical use and may be self-administered or given by a nonspecialist. There are 30 items with yes/no answers, and it takes about 8 to 10 minutes. Testing has been performed in nursing homes and with hospitalized patients, as well as community and office settings. Reliability and validity are considered good. Validity does decrease with increasing dementia. Sensitivity and specificity are quite good in relation to other screening tools (McDowell & Newell, 1996). Again, formal diagnoses of depression require clinical evaluation.

Hamilton Rating Scale for Depression. Created to measure the severity of depression in previously diagnosed patients, the Hamilton Rating Scale for Depression (HRSD) is designed to be applied by a clinician (Hamilton, 1960, 1967). Application time is at least 30 minutes and proceeds through 21 items by an essentially nonstructured interview in the original version. Revisions exist, including a structured version that can be applied by nonclinicians (Potts et al., 1990). The scale can distinguish severity of depression and is capable of detecting clinical change. Reliability and validity are considered good (McDowell & Newell, 1996). The scale has been used primarily in a research setting with depressed patients. The Carroll Rating Scale for Depression is a self-administered instrument based on the HRSD which can be used for screening and severity assessment (Carroll et al., 1981).

Montgomery-Åsberg Depression Rating Scale. The Montgomery-Åsberg Depression Rating Scale (MADRS) is designed to be sensitive to treatment effects in previously diagnosed patients (Montgomery & Åsberg, 1979). The focus of measurement is on the nonsomatic psychological and behavioral manifestations of depression, which may make it more appropriate than the HRSD for physically ill patients (McDowell & Newell, 1996). The 10 items are administered by a clinician, taking 20 to 60 minutes. It has been applied in inpatient and outpatient settings across a range of ages. Reliability and validity are both considered good (McDowell & Newell, 1996). Severity of depression cut-offs exist, although the primary purpose is to be sensitive to a change in clinical status.

Other depression scales. Several other depression scales exist, and no single comprehensive reference provides a quick review of all available scales. The scales selected for description above represent a range (from screening to detecting changes in the level of depressed symptomatology) of common measures, and they all have an established history of use. Two other prominent measures not discussed are the Zung Self-Rating Depression Scale, primarily used as a screening instrument (McDowell & Newell, 1996; Wilkin, Hallam, & Doggett, 1992; Zung, 1973) and the Hospital Anxiety and Depression Scale (Zigmond & Snaith, 1983), which is discussed under anxiety measures below. Investigators will need to turn to the original literature for final determination of appropriateness of a given measurement instrument.

Anxiety Scales

Anxiety as a construct for measurement is not yet well delineated. Generally speaking, anxiety is an unpleasant condition characterized by excessive and inappropriate worry and accompanied by typical physical symptoms. Of concern here will be generalized anxiety and not specific disease syndromes, such as phobic and panic disorders. The operationalization of anxiety has resulted in two separately measured concepts: anxiety as a trait—an enduring personality characteristic—and anxiety as a state—a transitory phenomenon (Kellner & Uhlenhuth, 1991; Walker, 1990). Each concept requires a different approach, with questions about trait referring to how a person feels generally, while state questions ask about present feelings. Most scales focus on psychological symptoms to avoid confusing results with symptoms of nonanxiety physical illness. In a related issue, anxiety is often accompanied by depression in clinical situations, and this can lead to difficulties in measuring either "pure" construct when a scale has items that are common to both conditions. Psychological stress is a related concept. Perhaps the most important conceptual difference is that anxiety, as a psychiatric disorder, is an inappropriate response, and may even exist without identifiable stressors. The effects of stress can be experienced by any person to any degree, depending on the intensity of environmental pressures. Anxiety affects well-being, and the physiological and psychological changes that result may increase susceptibility to illness or interfere with successful treatment. The health consequences of (nondisease state) anxiety are probably very similar to psychological stress. An interesting example of the direct impact of psychological stress on physical health was demonstrated by a study of susceptibility to the common cold. Healthy volunteers were exposed to respiratory viruses and quarantined. Increased rates of infection were observed in subjects with increased levels of measured stress (Cohen, Tyrrell, & Smith, 1991). Anxiety may affect compliance or choice of treatment as well.

Common measures often focus on psychological complaints, although there may be scales or items within scales that cover the somatic and behavioral manifestations of anxiety. Which manifestation is measured can be an advantage or disadvantage depending on the goals of the measurement. To detect all possible cases and rate their severity, all measures would be desirable. However, to avoid false positives in certain populations, such as patients with medical illnesses who have anxiety-like bodily symptoms, a concentration on the psychological aspects of anxiety would be better. Typical questions will be about things such as worry, agitation symptoms, and fright. The field of anxiety measures is not as fully developed as that of depression or social support. Two examples of established measures are briefly reviewed here.

Hospital Anxiety and Depression Scale. Designed as a self-assessment screening tool to detect states of anxiety and depression in hospital outpatient clinics, the Hospital Anxiety and Depression Scale (HAD) has eight items for anxiety and eight for depression (Zigmond & Snaith, 1983). The questions cover psychological rather than somatic complaints to avoid false positives from other medical illnesses. It takes about 20 minutes or less, and has been translated into foreign languages. The HAD has been used in a variety of medical patients in ages from 16 to 65 years. Validity appears good, although reliability is not as well documented (Wilkin et al., 1992).

State-Trait Anxiety Inventory. Originally developed to study the relationship between anxiety and learning, the State-Trait Anxiety Inventory (STAI) has been used in a variety of health care settings (Spielberger, Gorusch, & Lushene, 1970). It is self-administered and reportedly takes about 10 minutes to complete. There are 20 items on state and 20 items on trait anxiety. Foreign language translations and reference standards exist. The state questions could be used to monitor change, whereas the trait questions are more stable, as expected. Reliability is good. Validity appears good for the state component, although it has been questioned for the trait component, which might be measuring another dimension, such as dissatisfaction with self (Chaplin, 1984).

Other Anxiety Scales. For purposes of medical research in anxiety, the Hamilton Anxiety Scale may be considered, with its long history of use in the study of antianxiety drugs (Hamilton, 1959). It has been criticized as being nonspecific for anxiety (Kellner & Uhlenhuth, 1991). A complete review and discussion of anxiety scales does not exist at this time. Investigators looking for all existing options will need to turn to review articles and the original scale development reports.

Psychological Well-Being Scale

Psychological well-being occupies a position on the healthy side of the illness-to-wellness continuum. Measurement has been approached in different ways. One approach looks for fit between a person's current situation and his or her aspirations. Another probes feelings about daily experiences. A third focuses on detecting psychological distress (McDowell & Newell, 1996). Questions may also be directed toward a positive sense of complete psychological, social, and physical well-being. Items cover a broad range of areas, from feelings of loneliness, to contentment with appearance and energy level, to the occasional somatic symptom. Psychological questions are by far most common. Most scales are designed to discriminate degrees of wellness in a general sample of non-ill people, where measures of psychological morbidity would be insensitive to differences between people or changes in a person over time. The general nature of the items does not allow for specific diagnoses if poor psychological health is observed. Like general health measures, overall psychological well-being scales cast a broad net for detection of adverse mental health outcomes. Compared in Table 8–3 and reviewed in the text below are several established scales that represent a range of available measures.

Affect Balance Scale. The self-administered Affect Balance Scale (ABS) measures positive and negative affective responses to events of everyday life. It is designed for use in the general population as an indicator of current psychological well-being (Bradburn, 1969). There are 10 items and a yes/no format, so the test is brief. Reference standards exist from the Canadian Health Survey. Reliability and validity are both judged to be good (McDowell & Newell, 1996). Other more comprehensive scales exist, but the ABS has a long, established history of use, and its brevity could be a great advantage in a setting with time constraints.

General Well-Being Schedule. The General Well-Being Schedule (GWB) is an 18-item, self-administered questionnaire that covers energy level, health concerns, depression, and tension (Monk, 1981). The scale is intended for community surveys and was developed for the U.S. Health and Nutrition Examination Survey, the results of which provide reference standards. It is designed as a measure of general psychological well-being and distress, so it contains questions about positive and negative feelings. It takes about 10 minutes to complete. Reliability and validity are both considered very good, although the adequacy of

Table 8–3 Overview of Selected Psychological Well-Being Measures

Measurement Scale	Purpose	Population	Setting	Items/Time*
Affect Balance Scale (Bradburn, 1969)	Current psychological well-being	General	Population survey	10/Relatively brief
General Well-Being Schedule (Monk, 1981)	General psychological well-being and distress	General	Community survey	18/10 Min.
RAND Mental Health Inventory (Stewart et al., 1992; Viet & Ware, 1983)	Psychological distress and wellness in the healthy	General	Population survey	38/Relatively long
Life Satisfaction Index A (Neugarten, Havighurst, & Tobin, 1961)	General well-being	General older adults	Various clinical and community	20/Moderate
General Health Questionnaire (Goldberg, 1972)	Detection of psychiatric disorder	General, outpatients	Population survey, clincial	60/10 Min.

Note: All measures above are self-administered.

*Time measurement is not always published by the original authors nor available in published reviews of scales. When not available, a verbal estimate is based on the number of items, their content, and the response categories, relative to other similar scales.

test–retest reliability has been questioned, making assessment of individuals problematic (McDowell & Newell, 1996).

RAND Mental Health Inventory. Designed for population surveys, there are 38 items in the self-administered RAND Mental Health Inventory (MHI) (Stewart et al., 1992; Viet & Ware, 1983). Questions focus on affective states, including typical items used for anxiety and depression measurement, as well as questions about loss of control and positive affect. The goal was to produce a measure sensitive to psychological distress and wellness in generally healthy people. The test is relatively long, although a brief version has been evaluated (Berwick et al., 1991). Reliability and validity are both good (McDowell & Newell, 1996). The scale was used as the primary mental health outcome measure to predict health service use in the RAND Health Insurance Experiment (Viet & Ware, 1983).

Life Satisfaction Index. The Life Satisfaction (LSI) intends to measure general well-being in older adults, as conceptualized by zest, resolution, fortitude, congruence between achieved and desired goals, positive self-concept, and mood tone (Neugarten et al., 1961). It is applied to the general older adult population. The most commonly used version is the "A" index (LSIA), which contains 20 self-administered items. It has been used in a variety of settings, including different patient groups. A review of reliability and validity concludes that they are quite good, but there remains a question about whether this scale is measuring only the intended constructs and, if not, what else it measures (McDowell & Newell, 1996).

General Health Questionnaire. Created to detect nonpsychotic psychiatric disorders in medical consultations, the General Health Questionnaire (GHQ) also has been used extensively in outpatient clinical settings (Goldberg, 1972). The GHQ covers distress and symptoms of mood disorder, including somatic complaints. The full version has 60 items and takes about 10 minutes to complete; a shorter, 28-item version exists (Goldberg & Hillier, 1979), as does a user's guide to the different versions (Goldberg, 1978). Sensitivity and specificity are, on average, about 80% to 90%, and reliability and validity are both considered very good (McDowell & Newell, 1996). The scale has been used widely, and foreign language versions exist. It must be remembered that the measure is not intended to distinguish between or confirm psychiatric diagnoses, and its application is in screening for acute conditions rather than chronic.

Other psychological well-being scales. In addition to the above measures, other scales of general psychological well-being should be considered, depending on the theoretical model and research needs. The Philadelphia Geriatric Center Morale Scale, for example, provides an alternative (to the LSI) for assessment of generalized feeling of well-being in older adults (Lawton, 1975; McDowell & Newell, 1996). Investigators will need to extend their review beyond the measures briefly reviewed above to evaluate fully the choices among available measures. Because of the nonspecific nature of the psychological well-being measures, they are most appropriate as screening tools or group surveys.

Social Health Scales

Social health refers to the adequacy of social relationships; how they affect a person's well-being; and how they influence the risk, course, and outcomes of illness. Social relationships have long been associated with different incidence of disease. Prospective studies using variables representative of social network (marriage, contact with family and friends, church membership, group affiliation) have been independently and inversely associated with mortality rates in a variety of settings (House, Landis, & Umberson, 1988). The demographic variables of marriage, religiosity, and immigrant status may well mediate their effect through mechanisms that form the theoretical basis of social health measures. Social support has been associated with outcomes of disease. For example, emotional support was found to be independently related to risk of death over six months after an acute myocardial infarction in a prospective study of male and female older adult patients (Berkman, Leo-Summers, & Horowitz, 1992). In general, a good theoretical and empirical basis exists for five psychosocial factors that affect health: "1) major negative life events, 2) chronic stress, 3) lack of social relationships and supports, 4) lack of sense of control, efficacy, or mastery over one's work and life, and 5) high levels of hostility and/or mistrust in interpersonal relationships" (Kessler et al., 1995, p. 556–557). Clearly, there is some overlap between mental health, social health, and general psychological well-being. Reviewed here are the approaches taken with the more strictly "social" measures. Typical scale items will query the following areas: social contacts (frequency, quality, quantity), group participation, miscellaneous social activities (e.g., letter writing), work, finances, home, family, significant life events (e.g., divorce, retirement).

Social support has been the most studied component of social health. The primary theory holds that support networks buffer the effects of stressful life events that have adverse health consequences. Both the quantity and the quality of social networks can be measured. Another model of social health relies on the concept of successful social adjustment and role performance. A self-reported or independent observation of adjustment can be made. Both approaches have difficulty when we consider the following questions. What is the appropriate number and quality of social contacts for any given individual, considering personality differences and the different norms that people of different cultures and different ages within a culture all have? What defines *successful adjustment?* Don't role norms vary considerably over time and across regions? Measurement scales that contain questions about personal satisfaction with one's current network, adjustment, or role attempt to account for these differences in a model of person–environment fit (McDowell & Newell, 1996). Presumably, a person who has had a major change in his or her social network or life roles would respond to this type of measurement in a meaningful way. If no significant change has occurred, and a person is satisfied with his or her social functioning, one could argue that he or she should not be considered to have poor social health, even if the social relationships observed would be considered unsatisfactory or abnormal by most persons' standards. Additionally, it is not clear whether perceived or actual social support is more important. The former may affect one's sense of well-being with implications for improved outcomes, but the latter is necessary for direct care. Several examples of established scales that measure one or more theoretical dimensions of social health are compared in Table 8–4 and in the text below.

Norbeck Social Support Questionnaire. Developed to measure multiple quantitative and qualitative dimensions of an individual's social support network, the Norbeck Social Support Questionnaire (NSSQ) was designed for use in studies of health outcome (Norbeck et al., 1981). The measure inquires about practical support, such as financial and transportation assistance, as well as emotional support. There are 9 items, it is self-administered, and it takes about 10 minutes to complete. It has been applied in a variety of clinical situations, particularly among females, although it has also been used in an older adult, institutional population. Reliability and validity information is limited but appears good (Wilkin et al., 1992).

Social Relationship Scale. The Social Relationship Scale (SRS) was designed to assess the quantity and quality of an individual's social support network and the ways that social support cushions the effect of life stressors on health (McFarlane et al., 1981). It is self-administered and contains 6 items that correspond to areas of life such as home, work, and social events. The SRS is comprehensive in that it covers giving as well as receiving support. The scale was intended for use in studies of life events in general population samples. Reliability and validity measures appear acceptable, but information is limited (McDowell & Newell, 1996).

Social Support Questionnaire. The Social Support Questionnaire (SSQ) was designed to quantify the availability and satisfaction with social support for an individual (Sarason et al., 1987). Similar to the SRS, the SSQ asks for identification of individuals with whom the respondent interacts closely, then asks for a rating of the quality of that relationship. The full, 27-item version is self-administered and takes a long time relative to other similar scales, although an abbreviated 6-item version exists (Sarason et al., 1987). Reliability and validity are both good (McDowell & Newell, 1996). It is considered a good and generally applicable measure of social support.

Table 8–4 Overview of Selected Measures of Social Health

Measurement Scale	Purpose*	Population	Setting	Administration	Items/Time
Norbeck Social Support Questionnaire (Norbeck, Lindsey, & Carrieri, 1981)	Quantitative and qualitative dimensions of support in health outcomes	General clinical	Inpatient and outpatient, institutional	Self	9 Items/10 min.
Social Relationship Scale (McFarlane et al., 1981)	Extent and quality of support network for population research	General	Community	Self	6 Items/not reported
Social Support Questionnaire (Sarason et al., 1987)	Availability and satisfaction with support network for research	General	General	Self	27 Items/relatively long
Medical Outcomes Social Support Survey (Sherbourne & Stewart, 1991)	Availability and perception of support in chronic illness	Chronically ill, other potential	General	Self	20 items/relatively brief
Social Adjustment Scale (Weissman & Bothwell, 1976)	Social adjustment in depressed patients	Depressed, other potential	Outpatient, other	Self or interview	42 Items/self 15–20 min.; interview 45–60 min.

*Intent and use of the original measure. Other headings defined as in Table 8–2.

Medical Outcomes Study Social Support Survey. The Medical Outcomes Study Social Support Survey aims to cover five dimensions of social support: emotional support, informational support, tangible support, positive social interactions, and affection. Sherbourne and Stewart (1991) focused on the availability and perception of support rather than the number of individual relationships, as seen in other scales of similar intent. The scale has 20 items and is self-administered, taking a relatively brief amount of time to complete. The original population was chronically ill patients. Reliability and validity are considered very good, and the measure will probably prove to be more generally applicable with use over time (McDowell & Newell, 1996).

Social Adjustment Scale. The Social Adjustment Scale (SAS) was designed to evaluate the social adjustment outcomes of therapeutic interventions for psychiatric patients, although it is applicable in other populations (Weissman & Bothwell, 1976). The approach is to measure social adjustment through interpersonal relationships in a variety of roles, such as at work or within the family. There are 42 questions and two versions: a self-report and an interview. The self-report takes 15 to 20 minutes and the interview takes 45 to 60 minutes. Reliability and validity are considered quite good, and the measure does not appear to be affected by sociodemographic characteristics (McDowell & Newell, 1996). The scale is promising, therefore, for a variety of health outcomes assessments.

Other social well-being scales. Many other measures of social health exist, including social well-being subscales in mixed or general health status measures. Most scales are devoted to social health work with the concepts of social support, adjustment, or role functioning, although other theoretical approaches may arise in the future. There are other scales that demonstrate a different role from those reviewed above. For example, the Duke–University of North Carolina Functional Social Support Questionnaire has an advantage of being a brief, qualitative measure of functional aspects of social support, and it has been applied in a family practice clinic setting (Broadhead et al., 1988; McDowell & Newell, 1966; Wilkin et al., 1992). The Interview Schedule for Social Interaction (ISSI) is an in-depth, interview-based measure designed to assess the availability and supportive quality of relationships; it has been used primarily to research neurotic illness and assess outcomes of psychiatric care (Henderson, Byrne, & Duncan-Jones, 1981; McDowell & Newell, 1996). Again, selection of a scale for a specific research purpose requires a theoretical construct to determine the variables needed, familiarity with the original literature on scales of interest, and an up-to-date review of the evidence for their successful application.

Health Beliefs, Attitudes, and Behavior Scales

Health beliefs, attitudes, and behavior form a separate subsection that distinguishes scales that do not specifically aim to measure psychological or social health but still fall into the domain of psychological and social variables. These variables are concepts measured through scales that aim to quantify a specified characteristic of health beliefs and attitudes (about oneself or the health care system) or about health-related behavior (primarily the factors that determine behavior). The potential for impact on health care and outcomes will be argued through the conceptual model that drives the research. Some of these variables are compliance and motivation, culturally specific health beliefs, spirituality (discussed in part in the religiosity section of demographic variables), lifestyle issues (concerning diet, substance use, etc.), and perhaps many others, depending on one's point of view. Some of these areas will have formalized scale measures already developed; others will have been researched only through questionnaires or more informal information gathering.

Primarily for demonstration purposes, an example of measurement is discussed here for two important variables: personal health perceptions and motivation. Health perceptions, in terms of self-rated health, have been shown to be a good predictor of mortality (Idler & Kasl, 1991; Pijls, Feskens, & Kromhout, 1993). Motivation is a complex phenomenon of increasingly recognized significance given the strong behavioral component of chronic disease in industrialized nations.

Health Perceptions Questionnaire. The Health Perceptions Questionnaire (HPQ) was designed to survey people's perceptions of their own health, focusing on general assessment rather than the traditional components of physical, mental, and social health, and as a research instrument to explore health and illness behavior (Ware, 1976). It measures perception of past and current health, health outlook, susceptibility to illness, health worry, and attitude toward sickness and the sick role. The original measure contains 32 items, is self-administered, and takes about 7 minutes to complete. Alternative versions and reference standards exist (McDowell & Newell, 1996). Reliability and validity are both considered good (McDowell & Newell, 1996). The HPQ has been used to predict use of health services in populations and it has been applied in a clinical setting (Wilkin et al., 1992).

Self-Motivation Inventory. The Self-Motivation Inventory (SMI) was developed to provide an easily administered assessment of self-motivation, recognizing a need for a measure that might tie self-motivation to behavior and identify individuals who persevere or are prone to drop out of therapeutic programs (Dishman & Ickes, 1981). Questions involve personal perceptions about motivation and behavior. The measure is self-administered and has 40 items. It was originally used for adherence to an exercise program and subsequently has been used for weight loss programs. Its authors intend more extensive application. Validity appears good as does reliability in the original report, but, so far, its use has been too limited to draw broad conclusions.

CONCLUSION

Demographic, psychological, and social variables are important in outcomes research primarily because they influence a variety of outcomes. Some of these variables, such as depression, will be outcomes in their own right. The usefulness of these variables is often overlooked. The measurement of demographic variables appears deceptively simple but is actually complex. This occurs in part due to the difficulty in overcoming the natural tendency to conceptualize them in a simplistic manner. Additionally, the aggregate nature of many of these variables, such as socioeconomic status, means that multiple factors influencing health are involved in a single variable. These factors can be measured in different ways, and interpreting the mechanisms of their influence is complex. Variables should be carefully selected and measured to fulfill the needs of the study without overburdening data collection and analysis—a challenging task. It is the conceptual model (the theoretical framework that incorporates the hypothesis under question) that guides an investigator through variable selection and interpretation of results by specifying the relationship of the variables to the outcomes of interest.

Psychological and social variables are generally more complicated than demographic variables to measure because they are abstract concepts and must be operationalized into a practical measurement scale. There are diverse scales on a variety of measures in the literature, and finding the best one for a particular purpose takes effort. Scales may measure psychological, somatic, or behavioral dimensions of these variables, and there are advantages and disadvantages to measuring one or all of these dimensions. For example, measuring the dimension of somatic complaints with an anxiety scale can lead to a large number of false positives in a population of patients who have somatic symptoms from physical illness. For screening a population, measuring multiple dimensions of a concept is desirable to achieve a high sensitivity. Scales must be applicable to the population, setting, and expected range of responses. If the purpose is to measure change in a psychological or social variable, the scale must be sensitive to the level of change expected. If there is a good theoretical reason to apply a certain measure, but it has not been done in quite that setting or population before, it is generally advisable to use an existing measure rather than create a new one. Again, the conceptual model will help guide rational choices for measurement. If there is some factor a researcher would like to measure, chances are there is a device available just waiting to be applied.

REFERENCES

Abramson, J.H. (1990). *Survey methods in community medicine.* Singapore: Churchill Livingstone.

Andresen, E.M., Malmgren, J.A., Carter, W.B., & Patrick, D.L. (1994). Screening for depression in well older adults: Evaluation of a short form of the CES-D. *American Journal of Preventive Medicine, 10*(2), 77–84.

Beck, A.T., & Beck, R.W. (1972). Screening depressed patients in family practice: A rapid technique. *Postgraduate Medicine, 52*, 81–85.

Beck, A.T., Ward, C.H., Mendelson, M., Mock, J., & Erbaugh J. (1961). An inventory for measuring depression. *Archives of General Psychiatry, 4*, 561–571.

Berkman, L.F., Leo-Summers, L., & Horowitz, R.I. (1992). Emotional support and survival after myocardial infarction. *Annals of Internal Medicine, 117*, 1,003–1,009.

Berwick, D.M., Murphy, J.M., Goldman, P.A., Ware, J.E. Jr., Barsky, A.J., & Weinstein, M.C. (1991). Performance of a five-item mental health screening test. *Medical Care, 29*(2), 169–176.

Bradburn, N.M. (1969). *The structure of psychological well-being*. Chicago: Aldine.

Broadhead, W.E., Gehlbach, S.H., DeGruy, F.V., & Kaplan, B.H. (1988). The DUKE–UNC functional social support questionnaire. *Medical Care, 26*(7), 709–723.

Burman, N., & Margolin, G. (1992). Analysis of the association between marital relationships and health problems: An interactional perspective. *Psychological Bulletin, 112*(1), 39–63.

Carroll, B.J., Feinberg, M., Smouse, P.E., Rawson, S.G., & Greden, J.F. (1981). The Carroll rating scale for depression. I. Development, reliability, and validation. *British Journal of Psychiatry, 138*, 194–200.

Chandra, V., Szklo, M., Goldberg, R., & Tonascia, J. (1983). The impact of marital status on survival after an acute myocardial infarction: A population-based study. *American Journal of Epidemiology, 117*(3), 320–325.

Chaplin, W.F. (1984). State-trait anxiety inventory. In D.J. Keyser & R.C. Sweetland (Eds.), *Test critiques*, (vol. 1). Kansas City, MO: Test Corporation of America, 626–632.

Cockerham, W.C. (1986). *Medical sociology*. Englewood Cliffs, NJ: Prentice-Hall.

Cohen, S., Tyrrell, D.A.J., & Smith, A.P. (1991). Psychological stress and susceptibility to the common cold. *New England Journal of Medicine, 325*(9), 606–612.

Dishman, R.K., & Ickes, W. (1981). Self-motivation and adherence to therapeutic exercise. *Journal of Behavioral Medicine, 4*(4), 421–438.

Dohrenwend, B.P. (1990). Socioeconomic status (SES) and psychiatric disorders: Are the issues still compelling? *Social Psychiatry and Psychiatric Epidemiology, 25*, 41–47.

Dohrenwend, B.P., & Dohrenwend, B.S. (1976). Sex differences and psychiatric disorders. *American Journal of Sociology, 81*(6), 1,447–1,454.

Epstein, A.M., Stern, R.S., Tognetti, J., Begg, C.B., Hartley, R.M., Cumella, E., Jr., & Ayanian, J.Z., (1988). The association of patients' socioeconomic characteristics with the length of hospital stay and hospital charges within diagnosis-related groups. *New England Journal of Medicine, 318*(24), 1,579–1,585.

Fraser, G.E., Strahan, T.M., Sabate, J., Beeson, W.L., & Kissinger, D. (1992). Effects of traditional coronary risk factors on rates of incident: Coronary events in a low-risk population—the Adventist health study. *Circulation, 86*(2), 406–413.

Goldberg, D. (1978). *Manual of the general health questionnaire*. Windsor, England: NFER Publishing.

Goldberg, D.P. (1972). *The detection of psychiatric illness by questionnaire. Maudsley monograph no. 21*. London: Oxford University Press.

Goldberg, D.P., & Hillier, V.F. (1979). A scaled version of the general health questionnaire. *Psychological Medicine, 9*, 139–145.

Hamilton, M. (1959). The assessment of anxiety states by rating. *British Journal of Medical Psychology, 32*, 50–55.

Hamilton, M. (1960). A rating scale for depression. *Journal of Neurology, Neurosurgery, and Psychiatry, 23,* 56–62.

Hamilton, M. (1967). Development of a rating scale for primary depressive illness. *British Journal of Social and Clinical Psychology, 6,* 278–296.

Henderson, S., Byrne, D.G., & Duncan-Jones, P. (1981). *Neurosis and the social environment.* Sydney, Australia: Academic Press.

House, J.S., Landis, K.R., & Umberson, D. (1988). Social relationships and health. *Science, 241,* 540–545.

Idler, E.L., & Kasl, S. (1991). Health perceptions and survival: Do global evaluations of health status really predict mortality? *Journal of Gerontology, 46*(2), S55–S65.

Iezzoni, L. (Ed.). (1994). *Risk adjustment for measuring health care outcomes.* Ann Arbor, MI: Health Administration Press.

Joyce, C.R.B., Welldon, R.M.C., & Litt, B. (1965). The objective efficacy of prayer. *Journal of Chronic Disease, 18,* 367–377.

Kellner, R., & Uhlenhuth, E.H. (1991). The rating and self-rating of anxiety. *British Journal of Psychiatry, 159*(Suppl. 12), 15–22.

Kessler, R.C., House, J.S., Anspach, R.R., & Williams, D.R. (1995). Social psychology and health. In K.S. Cook, G.A. Fine, & J.S. House (Eds.), *Sociological perspectives on social psychology.* Needham Heights, MA: Allyn & Bacon, 548–570.

King, D.E., Hueston, W., & Rudy, M. (1994). Religious affiliation and obstetric outcome. *Southern Medical Journal, 87*(11), 1,125–1,128.

Lawton, M.P. (1975). The Philadelphia geriatric center morale scale: A revision. *Journal of Gerontology, 30*(1), 85–89.

Levin, J.S. (1994). Religion and health: Is there an association, is it valid, and is it causal? *Social Science and Medicine, 38*(11), 1,475–1,482.

Levin, J.S., & Vanderpool, H.Y. (1987). Is frequent religious attendance really conducive to better health? Toward an epidemiology of religion. *Social Science and Medicine, 24*(7), 589–600.

Liberatos, P., Link, B., & Kelsey, J.L. (1988). The measurement of social class in epidemiology. *Epidemiologic Reviews, 10,* 87–121.

Lyon, J.L., Gardner, K., & Gress, R.E. (1994). Cancer incidence among Mormons and non-Mormons in Utah (United States) 1971–85. *Cancer Causes and Control, 5,* 149–156.

Mausner, J.S., & Kramer, S. (1985). *Mausner & Bahn epidemiology—An introductory text.* Philadelphia: W.B. Saunders.

McDowell, I., & Newell, C. (1996). *Measuring health: A guide to rating scales and questionnaires.* New York: Oxford University Press.

McFarlane, A.H., Neale, K.A., Norman, G.R., Roy, R.G., & Streiner, D.L. (1981). Methodological issues in developing a scale to measure social support. *Schizophrenia Bulletin, 7,* 90–100.

Mendes de Leon, C.F., Appels, A.W.P.M., Otten, F.W.J., & Schouten, E.G. (1992). Risk of mortality and coronary heart disease by marital status in middle-aged men in the Netherlands. *International Journal of Epidemiology, 21*(3), 460–466.

Monk, M. (1981). Blood pressure awareness and psychological well-being in the Health and Nutrition Examination Survey. *Clinical Investigations in Medicine, 4,* 183–189.

Montgomery, S.A., & Åsberg, M. (1979). A new depression scale designed to be sensitive to change. *British Journal of Psychiatry, 134,* 382–389.

Morris, J.N., & Heady, J.A. (1953a). Coronary heart-disease and physical activity of work: Part 1. *Lancet, 21,* 1,053–1,057.

Morris, J.N., & Heady, J.A. (1953b). Coronary heart-disease and physical activity of work: Part 2. *Lancet, 28,* 1,111–1,120.

Navarro, V. (1991). Race or class or race and class: Growing mortality differentials in the United States. *International Journal of Health Services, 21*(2), 229–235.

Neale, A.N., Tilley, B.C., & Vernon, S.W. (1986). Marital status, delay in seeking treatment, and survival from breast cancer. *Social Science and Medicine, 23*(3), 305–312.

Neugarten, B.L., Havighurst, R.J., & Tobin, S.S. (1961). The measurement of life satisfaction. *Journal of Gerontology, 16,* 134–143.

Norbeck, J.S., Lindsey, A.M., & Carrieri, V.L. (1981). The development of an instrument to measure social support. *Nursing Research, 30*(5), 264–269.

Pijls, L.T.J., Feskens, E.J.M., & Kromhout, D. (1993). Self-rated health, mortality, and chronic diseases in elderly men. *American Journal of Epidemiology, 138*(10), 840–848.

Pol, L.G., & Thomas, R.K. (1992). *The demography of health and health care.* New York: Plenum Press.

Potts, M.K., Daniels, M., Bernam, M.A., & Wells, K.B. (1990). A structured interview version of the Hamilton depression rating scale: Evidence of reliability and versatility of administration. *Journal of Psychiatric Research, 24*(4), 335–350.

Radloff, L.L. (1977). The CES-D scale: A self-report depression scale for research in the general population. *Applied Psychological Measurement, 1,* 385–401.

Sarason, I.G., Sarason, B.R., Shearin, E.N., & Pierce, G.R. (1987). A brief measure of social support: Practical and theoretical implications. *Journal of Social and Personal Relationships, 4,* 497–510.

Sherbourne, C.D., & Stewart, A.L. (1991). The MOS social support survey. *Social Science and Medicine, 32,* 705–714.

Sherrill, K.A., & Larson, D.B. (1988). Adult burn patients: The role of religion in recovery. *Southern Medical Journal, 81*(7), 821–825.

Shryock, H.S., Siegel, J.S., & associates. (1976). *The methods and materials of demography.* San Diego, CA: Academic Press.

Spielberger, C.D., Gorusch, R.L., & Lushene, R.E. (1970). *Manual for the state-trait anxiety inventory.* Palo Alto, CA: Consulting Psychologists Press.

Stewart, A.L., Ware, J.E.J., Sherbourne, C.D., & Wells, K.B. (1992). Psychological distress/well-being and cognitive functioning measures. In A.L. Stewart & J.E.J. Ware (Eds.), *Measuring functioning and well-being: The medical outcomes study approach.* Durham, NC: Duke University Press, 102–142.

U.S. Public Health Service. (1987). *National health interview survey questionnaire.* Hyattsville, MD: National Center for Health Statistics, Division of Health Interview Statistics.

U.S. Public Health Service, Health Care Financing Administration. (1980). *The International Classification of Diseases, 9th Revision, Clinical Modification.* PHS 80-1,260. Washington, DC: Author.

Verbrugge, L.M. (1979). Marital status and health. *Journal of Marriage and the Family, 41,* 267–285.

Verbrugge, L.M. (1989). The twain meet: Empirical explanations of sex differences in health and mortality. *Journal of Health and Social Behavior, 30,* 282–304.

Viet, C.T., & Ware, J.E.J. (1983). The structure of psychological distress and well-being in general populations. *Journal of Consulting and Clinical Psychology, 51,* 730–742.

Walker, L.G. (1990). The measurement of anxiety. *Postgraduate Medicine, 66*(suppl. 2), S11–S17.

Ware, J.E. (1976). Scales for measuring general health perceptions. *Health Services Research, 11,* 396–415.

Weissman, J.S., Gastsonis, C., & Epstein, A.M. (1992). Rates of avoidable hospitalization by insurance status in Massachusetts and Maryland. *JAMA, 268*(17), 2,388–2,394.

Weissman, M.M., & Bothwell, S. (1976). Assessment of social adjustment by patient self-report. *Archives of General Psychiatry, 33*, 1,111–1,115.

Wilkin, D., Hallam, L., & Doggett, M. (1992). *Measurement of need and outcome for primary health care*. New York: Oxford University Press.

Yesavage, J.A., & Brink, T.L. (1983). Development and validation of a geriatric depression screening scale: A preliminary report. *Journal of Psychiatric Research, 17*(1), 37–49.

Zigmond, A.S., & Snaith, R.P. (1983). The hospital anxiety and depression scale. *Acta Psychiatrica Scandinavica, 67*, 361–370.

Zung, W.W.K. (1973). From art to science: The diagnosis and treatment of depression. *Archives of General Psychiatry, 29*, 328–337.

Part IV_____

Technical and Practical Issues

Measurement is a central part of all aspects of outcomes work. It is discussed in a separate chapter because the principles involved can be applied to all the other components of the basic outcomes equation. The form of a measure and its psychometric properties are worthy of concern, but one should not become so absorbed in the details of psychometrics that one forgets the main measurement goal: to measure what is important, not what is easy. As measures have been developed, they have become more sophisticated, and the audience reading outcomes studies or proposals has begun to demand strong pedigrees for these measures. It, therefore, makes good sense to use an established, tested measure whenever possible rather than trying to create one from scratch. The chapter on measurement attempts to provide a buyer's guide to this complex topic. It addresses both basic issues and the implications for measurement of some of the newer, more sophisticated modeling methods.

The book closes with a string of observations and suggestions about various aspects of outcomes research, including data quality, analytic issues, and ethical considerations. Practical tips are mixed with more philosophic discussions. To provide a tangible context, an example is presented of how an outcomes study was developed and conducted.

9

Measurement

Jennifer Frytak

CHAPTER OUTLINE

- What Is Measurement?
- How Can Measures Be Conceptualized?
- What Is the Best Information Source?
- How Are Characteristics of an Object Turned into Numbers?
- Weighting/Aggregation: How Are Items in a Measure Combined?
- How Useful Is the Measure?
- How Can a Measure's Sensitivity to Change Be Assessed?
- How Are Changes in Health Status Measures Interpreted?
- How Do Multiple- Versus Single-Item Measures Compare?
- What Are the Shortcomings of Traditional Multiple-Item Scales?
- What about Measurement Error?

Measurement is fundamental to conducting health outcomes research. Making sense of clinical, social, and economic observations requires some method of quantifying them. While measurement of these factors is a regular occurrence, poor measurement has been an ongoing problem in conducting outcomes research. Measurement of variables of interest is linked to all steps of the scientific process: conceptualization of the study, analysis of the data, and interpretation of the results. One's measures are only as good as one's conceptualization of the concept, one's data are only as good as one's measures, and one's results are only as good as one's data.

Designing an outcomes study involves two critical steps: (1) conceptualization and (2) operationalization of the variables of interest. The conceptual model can be based on prior empirical work or driven by theory. The conceptual model should display the relationships between the outcomes of interest and the factors expected to influence these outcomes. The model will drive the analysis plan. The model becomes a road map for both the data collection and the analysis phases of the study. It is a useful tool to organize concepts, hypotheses, and timing of interventions and to clarify the purpose of the study.

In the second step, measurement is used to quantify the conceptual model. *Operationalizing* variables involves specifying the assumptions that translate theoretical/conceptual variables into empirical ones (i.e., measurement). When specifying these assumptions, it is useful to have a conceptual model of the variable one is trying to measure, especially if the variable is complex. For example, different conceptual models of health-related quality of life result in different dimensions of health being measured. The investigators must describe the data source for each variable in the study (e.g., survey, claims data, record review, etc.), the level of aggregation for each variable (e.g., continuous or categorical), and the specific measures for each variable. Existing measures for the variables may be available or new ones may need to be developed.

Achieving a good balance between conceptualization and measurement is a challenge in any study. The two steps are necessarily linked, but one runs the risk of focusing too heavily on one step and neglecting the other. On the one hand, an investigator may develop a wonderful theory on the role of psychosocial factors in achieving desirable outcomes for patients with congestive heart failure but then rely on easily available proxy variables for psychosocial factors to test his or her hypotheses. In this scenario, if the proxy variables do not measure well what they are supposed to measure, the investigator will not be able to provide adequate evidence to test the theory. On the other hand, investigators often assume that they can measure anything that they can give a name to without much thought to an underlying conceptual model for developing the measure (Duncan, 1984). It is possible that several different investigators will develop substantively different measures of disability, but by name, each will be measuring the same thing. It is easy to see the potential problems of generalizing findings on disability across research studies. Of course, in practice, one may be reduced to using crude measures to take the first crack at a particular problem, such as analyzing an unanticipated insight from one's data set. Overall, a good rule of thumb is that researchers should not attempt to measure something that they cannot conceptualize nor should they use a measure that they are not able to analyze correctly.

WHAT IS MEASUREMENT?

Measurement is an easy concept to visualize but a difficult one to define simply. Commonly, it is defined as the assignment of numbers to characteristics of objects, events, or people according to rules (Stevens, 1981). Investigators attempt to map numbers onto a set of objects so that the numbers represent the underlying relationships between the objects (Pedhazur & Schmelkin, 1991). For example, a ruler is used to measure the lengths of two pieces of string. The ruler assigns a number to each length, say 4 inch and 8 inch. Using this method, it is possible to state numerically that one string is half the length of the other. This provides a numeric description of the attribute. Imagine how difficult it would be in clinical or any other research if researchers had to rely strictly on verbal descriptions of characteristics of objects as a means for comparisons among the objects.

When choosing existing measures or developing new ones, it is important to keep in mind that all measurement is imperfect for two reasons:

1. Anything investigators measure is an abstraction from reality.
2. Anything measured is measured with error.

One can never measure anything directly. Instead, particular features or attributes of an object, person, or phenomenon are measured (Nunnally & Bernstein, 1994). For example, researchers do not measure an older woman, per se, but they may measure her functional disability. Recognizing that it is attributes that are measured emphasizes that any measurement is an abstraction from "reality." Realistically, researchers often end up sacrificing richness of a construct for a quantifiable and generalizable measure. Other than her ability to function, little information on this older woman is captured. In fact, even the information on functioning may be incomplete, since unknown features of her environment may dramatically affect what she physically *can* do and what she *does* do. Also, since researchers are constrained to using man-made instruments and protocols to measure attributes of an object or person, all measurements are subject to error, even in the most controlled situations. Inherently, measurement is an indirect process, since researchers are confined to their senses (or, at most, extensions of them) (Blalock & Hubert, 1982).

Historically, clinicians have been most confident measuring observable physical attributes of patients. However, in the current environment of outcomes research, many of the attributes of interest are not observable (e.g., quality of life and patient satisfaction). Phenomena such as quality of life, functional disability, depression, and even diseases like coronary artery disease, diabetes, or Alzheimer's disease can be thought of as latent constructs. *Latent constructs* are abstract ideas formulated by the clinician or investigator to explain certain phenomena that are observed in a clinical setting or elsewhere. Measuring latent constructs seems even more indirect than measuring observable attributes, since the clinician will never be able to confirm absolutely the former's existence. For example, a clinician has confidence in a given diagnosis only to the degree that the patient's symptoms are consistent with his or her experience with the disease. Similarly, the clinician's confidence in measuring body temperature with a thermometer is based on experience of accurate readings with the given thermometer and his or her competence in using the thermometer. Physical attributes are often measured as indicators of a latent construct such as disease. For example, blood sugar levels are associated with a complex series of metabolic processes that constitute diabetes mellitus. (Even blood sugar measurements are not direct; they rely on indirect chemical reactions that produce color changes.)

Everyday clinical practice relies on many latent constructs and involves the measurement of both observable and unobservable phenomena. Measuring the magnitude of latent constructs often involves constructing a scale. Researchers assume that the strength of the latent construct in each individual causes each item in a scale to take on a given value (DeVellis, 1991). An individual who has trouble functioning independently should score higher on a functional disability scale than a person who has no trouble functioning. Measuring observable physical attributes relies on a properly calibrated medical instrument or machine such as a thermometer or a blood pressure cuff. It is common when measuring physical properties—both physical attributes solely or those as indicators of a latent construct—to gain a false sense of security that one is accurately measuring what one intends to measure. Clinicians and investigators are more wary of a measurement based on scales. For example, they may have less confidence in a level of depression obtained by the Geriatric Depression Scale than a measurement of blood pressure obtained by a health professional using a blood pressure cuff. However, if one considers all the opportunities for conceptualization and measurement error when measuring either observable or unobservable phenomena, accepting any type of measurement involves taking a leap of faith. Consider the following example.

Measuring blood pressure generally involves many approximations. The force used to constrict an arm is considered to reflect the pressure in a blood vessel. Careful study suggests that this relationship can be influenced by a number of factors. For example, the circumference of the arm affects the force needed to constrict the artery. Different cuff sizes influence this relationship. The circumstances around making the blood pressure determinations can produce substantial results. Some people may experience higher blood pressures because of the anxiety induced by a visit to the doctor. Dramatic improvements can occur simply by having someone else take the measurement in a more informal setting. In truth, blood pressure determinations are samples of a parameter that varies widely. Careful studies of blood pressure measured periodically over a 24-hour period show wide fluctuations for the same person. Clearly, the single determination of blood pressure at a given point in time is but a pale imitation of the complex physical phenomenon it represents.

Measurement is a complex task, and several issues need to be considered when either choosing a measurement scale to include in a study or developing a new scale for a study. The construct of functional disability and handicap is used here as an illustrative example to demonstrate the variety of measurement approaches and issues investigators have tackled to capture the idea of functional disability. Scales of this type are generally described as activities of daily living (ADL) scales and instrumental activities of daily living (IADL) scales. ADLs address basic tasks that are needed for independent living; IADLs deal with somewhat more complex tasks needed to maintain an independent lifestyle in the community.

No single approach to the measurement of any construct is universally accepted. This is evident from the sheer number of ADL and IADL scales available for use. McDowell and Newell (1996) reviewed over 50 ADL scales and chose to include 6 in their book. These scales differ in a number of dimensions: content, metric, method of scoring, length, method of administration, and rigor of determining their reliability and validity. Given these circumstances, these scales would not likely yield similar scores of disability or be easily comparable.

HOW CAN MEASURES BE CONCEPTUALIZED?

First, researchers should determine clearly what it is that they want to measure and how the information will be used. Theory and the conceptual model can serve as guides to decide how broad or narrow the measure needs to be in several respects.

1. **Is it intended as a generic or disease-specific measure?** (For a complete discussion of this issue, see the chapters on generic and disease-specific outcomes measures.) For instance, an investigator may be interested in disability in a nursing home population. Initially, it seems that a generic measure may serve the study well. However, if the study question specifically deals with disability of arthritis patients in nursing homes, a disease-specific measure may also be considered.

2. **What is the scope of the measure?** The content of different disability scales varies widely. The following topics have appeared in disability scales: self-care, mobility, travel, body movement, home management, medical condition, senses, mental capacity, work, resources, social interaction, hobbies, communication, and behavior problems (McDowell & Newell, 1996). One could choose several of these items or all of them.

3. **What level of precision is needed from the measure for the study?** This question often involves both responsiveness to change and concerns about floor and ceiling effects. For example, using the functional disability questions from the Sickness Impact Profile (SIP) to capture changes in functioning in a well older adult population may be a mistake since the SIP has been

shown to differentiate well between those with poor health but not well between states in basically healthy older adults (Andresen et al., 1995). This represents a *ceiling effect:* an inability to demonstrate improvement. Similarly, the ADL scale would be a bad choice to measure functioning in a well population, since it generally measures a range of very low functioning. A *floor effect* is an inability to demonstrate deterioration (i.e., measure a trait below a given range).

Well-articulated goals for the chosen measure will help ensure the quality of the data obtained. For example, in terms of disability measures, it should be clear whether one is interested in what an individual does versus what an individual can do (Young et al., 1996). Likewise, specific scales may be conceptually inappropriate for certain populations. A scale used for assessing depression in younger adults may not be appropriate for assessing depression in older adults and vice versa. Questions about physical symptoms related to depression in adults may reflect normative health changes in older adults. Scales developed to measure disability in a younger, developmentally disabled population may include items addressing work-force issues that are not applicable to retired older adults. Too often, scales take on an artificial reality after they have been in use for awhile, and people assume that they are applicable to any study population.

Finally, it is important to be aware of the analysis requirements of the study before data collection of the measures is undertaken. The data source for each variable and any problems with the quality or availability of the data should be clear in advance. It is useful to make dummy tables that lay out how each variable will be used in the analysis phase. The format of the tables will vary depending on whether the variables are continuous or categorical. Continuous variables such as temperature or expenditures can take on any numerical value. "A continuous variable is one in which objects differ in degree, not in kind. . . . A categorical variable is a classificatory variable on which objects classified differ in kind, not degree" (Pedhazur & Schmelkin, 1991, pp. 175–176).

WHAT IS THE BEST INFORMATION SOURCE?

When choosing an already developed measure, certain issues must be considered. In some cases there may be a choice between using a report and making a direct measure of performance. The former usually addresses what is typically done, whereas the latter tests performance under controlled conditions (Hoeymans et al., 1996). Measures taken off the shelf have been developed for a specific information source with particular respondents in mind. The respondent may be the patient, the clinician, or some other proxy. Usually, the decision is based on who will be the most accurate source of information for the characteristic of interest. The effects of relying on proxies vary with the type of information sought. Proxies cannot be expected to have insight into all areas, such as pain. Most items from a medical history can be reliably obtained from proxies (assuming the proxy has had sufficient opportunity to observe the patient), but some cannot (Weiss et al., 1996).

Historically, medicine has overlooked patient input and relied heavily on physician judgment. However, in many cases, physicians get their information from the patients. Passing the information through an extra filter may make it more or less accurate. Research has shown that proxies of older adults tend to report lower functioning than the older adults themselves (Magaziner et al., 1988; Rubenstein et al., 1984). Each type of respondent has his or her own perspective; it is important to be aware of the characteristics of the information source that may bias the results or inhibit getting the necessary information. Using a standardized form loses the richness of information obtained; a general depression scale does not capture all the unique details of Mrs. Smith's situation. This loss is offset by the ability to quantify and compare information across patients. A certain level of cautious skepticism about established measures is useful. Many established scales have been developed on the basis of expert opinion; it is possible that they are building on past misconceptions rather than measuring what was intended.

HOW ARE CHARACTERISTICS OF AN OBJECT TURNED INTO NUMBERS?

Once investigators understand what variables they are interested in studying, they must decide how the variable will be quantified. The term *scaling* refers to how they assign numbers to the characteristics of the objects they are measuring. Each variable in the study must be scaled. (See Table 9–1.) Some variables are scales that consist of a single item, whereas other, often more complex, variables are scales that consist of an aggregation of multiple items. For a single-item scale or for each single item in a multiple-item scale, the response set must be scaled. The *response set* is the choice set that the respondent has for answering a given question. The response set determines the type of scale. With multiple-item scales, both the choice of response set and aggregation of the individual items determine the type of scale. Typically, variables are either *categorical* or *continuous*. This is a helpful dichotomy to apply to scales, since the type of scale will determine the eventual statistical procedures that can be used with the scale. Following are four types of measurement scales (Stevens, 1981):

1. **As a single item, the *nominal measure* has a categorical response set with no particular ordering.** Numbers are used as labels in order to classify objects into distinct categories; all objects can fit into only one category, and

Table 9–1 Types of Measurement Scales

Scale	Aggregation	Example of Response Set
Nominal	Categorical	Gender: female=1, male=0
Ordinal	Categorical	Can you dress and undress? 1) yes, without difficulty 2) yes, with minor difficulty 3) yes, with major difficulty 4) no, not able to
Interval	Continuous	How much difficulty do you have dressing and undressing? No difficulty _____ Unable to dress alone
Ratio	Continuous	$\dfrac{5 \text{ ft.}}{4 \text{ ft.}} = \dfrac{60 \text{ in.}}{48 \text{ in.}}$

every object must fit into a category. Classification is prevalent in outcomes research. Examples of nominal measures include: gender, race, hospital type, and diagnosis-related groups (DRGs). A simple yes/no question would be a nominal level measure.

2. **As a single item, the *ordinal measure* has an ordered categorical response set.** Numbers are used to represent a rank ordering between a set of objects given a particular attribute. Distances between the objects are not equal and cannot be meaningfully interpreted. An example of an ordinal measure would be an ADL question on dressing: Can you dress and undress? (1) yes, without difficulty, (2) yes, with minor difficulty, (3) yes, with major difficulty, (4) no, not able to. The distance between minor difficulty and no difficulty is not necessarily the same as the distance between minor and major difficulty.

3. **As a single item, the *interval measure* has a continuous response set.** The distance between each category is assumed to be the same (i.e., the numbers can be meaningfully interpreted). An example of an interval-level scale would be a visual analog scale. To obtain an interval-level response, one could have respondents mark their levels of difficulty dressing and undressing on a line of fixed length. No difficulty and inability to dress oneself alone anchor the line.

4. **The *ratio measure* is an interval measure with a true zero.** An example of a ratio measure would be height. There is a true zero, and, when the unit of

measurement changes, the ratio still stays the same. A child who is 5 feet tall is 1.25 times taller than one who is 4 feet tall. The ratio of these two heights stays the same when converted to inches. *Magnitude estimation* is a process believed to yield ratio-level scores. Suppose bathing is assigned as the benchmark ADL with a score of 500. Raters would then assign a weight of 250 to an ADL that contributed half as much to overall dependency.

The choice of measure implies the range of acceptable statistics to use with the measure. Parametric statistics (regression, averages, etc.) are inappropriate for nominal and ordinal (categorical) measures but appropriate for interval- and ratio-level (continuous) measures. Nominal and ordinal measures should be analyzed using nonparametric statistics. Table 9–1 shows the relationships between these types of measures. A good rule of thumb is to collect continuous data, or at least not dichotomous data, as often as possible. For some analyses, a mean change is less meaningful than the proportion that moves from one category to the other, but it is easier to categorize or establish a cut-off point post hoc. Depending on what a patient's baseline blood pressure measure was, a 10-millimeter change may mean different things. Dichotomous measures require larger sample sizes to demonstrate an effect and are less reliable than continuous measures (Streiner & Norman, 1995).

To measure the magnitude of continuous underlying attributes, several techniques are used: rating scales, comparative methods, magnitude estimation, and econometric methods. Using *rating scales*, the magnitude of an attribute is estimated by asking the respondent about the characteristic directly, using such tools as a visual analog scale or a Likert scale. Likert-type scales involve summing individual responses to a set of questions on an agree–disagree continuum (e.g., strongly agree, agree, disagree, strongly disagree) to calculate a score of disability. The response set is symmetric. Scale values are not assigned to individual items; only the total score is scalable. While individual items in the Likert scale are ordinal, total scores are treated as interval by most investigators and do not introduce substantial bias (Nunnally & Bernstein, 1994), as long as the scale is measuring only one underlying characteristic. Disputes on constructing the Likert scale arise around issues such as the appropriate number of categories and the use of an odd or even number of categories. The number of categories generally ranges from 5 to 9. Likert-based scaling methods are widely used, since they are inexpensive to design, easy to understand, and easy to administer.

Comparative methods involve an initial scaling of items on an interval-level scale (usually calibrating to a normal distribution) by a group of judges prior to obtaining actual responses. Items are scaled by either asking the judges to rank a large number of statements from most favorable to least favorable or to compare each item to each other item to distinguish which of the pair has more of the attributes in question. After the scale has been calibrated, a respondent chooses which statements apply to him or her; scores of individual items are aggregated by summing or averaging. These methods guarantee interval-level data, but scale construction is expensive and difficult and does not guarantee measurement of a single, underlying construct or unbiased rankings by the judges (McIver & Carmines, 1981).

Most of the early functional disability scales relied on another comparative method, the *Guttman scaling approach*. This type of scale is hierarchical and deterministic in nature, and measurement of a single, underlying construct of interest is required (Nunnally & Bernstein, 1994). Given the hierarchical nature of the scale, developmentally oriented constructs, such as ADLs, (e.g., bathing, dressing, transferring, toileting, feeding) work best with this method of scaling. Katz et al. (1963) developed a scale of ADLs based on the assumption that one loses and gains functions in a certain order (hierarchical). If one is dependent at Functional Level 3, one is necessarily dependent at Levels 1 and 2. *Deterministic models* of scaling assume no measurement error. Each score on the scale indicates the exact pattern of responses about the respondent's dependence. In practice, coefficients of stability and reproducibility are used to determine the degree of deviation from perfect ordering in the respondents of the sample. Finding constructs suitable for use with the Guttman method is difficult, and the data obtained are ordinal. Even the ADL construct has proven problematic. Research conducted with a sample of Medicaid-eligible, disabled older adults and a national sample of noninstitutionalized older adults shows that many hierarchical patterns of dependency other than the Katz method are possible (Lazaridis et al., 1994; Travis & McAuley, 1990). The common practice of using simple counts of ADLs assumes a hierarchy, equal weighting of each ADL in the count, and interval-level properties. These assumptions are somewhat tenuous.

In an effort to move beyond ordinal properties and equal weighting assumptions of standard measures, various scaling techniques have been used to weight health or dependency states. Recently, magnitude estimation techniques were used to obtain a weighted ratio-level scale of functional dependency (Finch, Kane, & Philp, 1995). In magnitude estimation, a reference item from a given construct is chosen and given a scale value. All remaining items are rated numerically with respect to how similar or dissimilar each is from the reference item. Using bathing as the standard (500), members of an expert panel each rated 13 function domains based on their judgment of how much the need for human assistance to perform the function contributes to overall dependency. The panel members then assigned weights from 0 to 100 to the level of assistance (e.g., a little assistance, a lot of assistance, complete assistance) needed to perform the functional activity. Average weights were then assigned for each ADL.

Since the scale exhibits ratio-level properties, a composite score is calculated. Finch et al. (1995) found that their scale was more sensitive to the nature and extent of functional losses in older adults than simple counts of ADLs and IADLs.

Their scale did not assume equal weight and did not arbitrarily dichotomize level of dependency for the ADLs and IADLs.

Cost-effectiveness analysis in health care has sparked the development of various utility (preference) measures of health care quality. A numerical value is assigned to health states with 1 for a healthy state and 0 for dead. Weights for each state can be determined by aggregating responses from a variety of scaling methods, including rating scales and magnitude estimation, but economists favor the standard gamble or time trade-off methods that are based on economic theory (Kaplan, 1995). The *standard gamble* asks the respondent to choose between an outcome that is certain but less than ideal or gamble on an outcome that is uncertain but leads to either perfect health or death given set probabilities. (See Figure 9–1.) The *time trade-off* method discards the difficult concept of probabilities and offers respondents a choice between perfect health for a set amount of time or less-than-perfect health for a variable amount of time. Economists argue that aggregation is more plausible using these methods in comparison to rating scales with ordinal-level properties. However, these methods assume rational decision making on the part of the respondents. Research suggests that this is not necessarily the case (Tversky & Kahneman, 1981). Researchers have found that these methods are difficult for respondents to understand and time-consuming to administer (Streiner & Norman, 1995).

WEIGHTING/AGGREGATION: HOW ARE ITEMS IN A MEASURE COMBINED?

For multi-item scales, once investigators understand how the responses in the questions are scaled, they need to think about how the items in the scale are combined. A common way to combine the items is to add them. However, simply adding the items may obscure important assumptions. One is assuming the weights for each item as well as the metric. Adding up the scale items assumes that each item contributes equally to the total score. However, the choice of a response set may inadvertently weight the items. Assume that one response set is 1 2 3 4 5. Choosing a response set of 1 3 5 7 9 for a different item assumes that the highest response of the latter set is 9 times greater than the lowest response, whereas in the first set, it was only 5 times greater. Also, one should only aggregate items that measure a single underlying construct. Apples and oranges should not be added together; it is not appropriate to combine several different constructs into a single score. Inadvertent weighting is possible if different aspects of a single construct are measured with different numbers of items. For instance, if an overall measure of functional disability had three questions dealing with self-care and five questions dealing with mobility, mobility would be weighted more heavily in the overall score. In combining subscales, this unintentional weighting should be

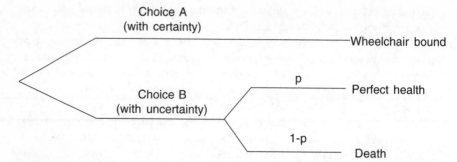

Figure 9–1 Standard Gamble Method. *Source:* Based on G. Torrance and D. Feeny, Utilities and Quality-Adjusted Life Years, *International Journal of Technology Assessment in Health Care*, Vol. 5, No. 4, pp. 559–575, © 1989.

corrected for by dividing the subscale score by the number of items in the subscale (i.e., using the averages of the subscales). Unintentional weighting in scales can also occur if items in a scale are very highly correlated. Thus, a high score on Question 2 would lead to high scores on items highly correlated with Question 2, giving certain aspects of the underlying construct extra weight.

Careful consideration of the cut-point in a response set is also important since it will dramatically affect the overall level of the construct measured in a given population. For example, suppose a researcher wants to do a simple count of disabilities, and the response categories are these: without help from someone, with a little help from someone, and with a lot of help from someone. Defining *disability* as doing something with a lot of help results in not capturing the part of the population that has moderate levels of disability for one's research study.

To weight a scale, researchers can derive the weights empirically or theoretically. *Theoretical weights* are chosen by the researcher based on his or her knowledge of the underlying characteristic. Certain scale items may be thought to contribute more heavily to the measurement of the characteristic. *Empirical weights* are often the coefficients from a multiple regression of total score on the individual items in the scale, or the item-total correlations (scale item = total score) can be used as the weights. Generally, the regression weights are unstable across samples due to large sampling errors, and much evidence suggests that weighting makes little difference, especially when scales contain at least 20 items (Nunnally & Bernstein, 1994). However, there is some evidence to the contrary if the number of scale items are small, and the items in the scale are relatively heterogeneous (Streiner & Norman, 1995). Functional status measures may benefit from weighting given the heterogeneity of the items (bathing, toileting, dressing) covered in these scales. Weighted or unweighted, once the total score has been calculated, it is important to be able to compare scores across similar scales. The best method is to transform the total score of each scale into a normalized, standardized score (Streiner & Norman, 1995).

HOW USEFUL IS THE MEASURE?

An important part of selecting a measure for use in a study is establishing the usefulness of the measure. Traditionally, this process involves assessing the reliability and validity of a measure. Assessing *reliability* involves showing that measurement is performed in a reproducible manner. Assessing *validity* means measuring what one intended to measure. A scale that always overweighs patients by exactly 10 pounds is an example of a reliable scale but not a valid one. Conversely, if the scale randomly overweighed and underweighed patients, the scale would be unreliable and invalid. Reliability is a necessary, but not sufficient, condition for validity.

As noted earlier, measurement is always subject to error. Measurement error lies at the heart of reliability and validity. One way to think about error in a measure is as *random* and *nonrandom measurement error*. Reliability is largely a function of random error that is completely unsystematic in nature. Random error could be caused by such things as keypunch and coding errors, ambiguous instructions, interviewer mistakes, or inconsistent responses. As random error in the measure increases, the reliability of the measure decreases. Validity is largely a function of nonrandom measurement error or systematic error. Nonrandom error generally occurs when a measure is measuring more than one construct or when the method of collecting the data systematically biases the results (Carmines & Zeller, 1979; Maruyama, in press).

A common misperception is that once the reliability and validity of a measure have been established, they are no longer an issue when the measure is used in future studies. This is false, since measurement error is inherent to a particular sample; reliability and validity are artifacts of the given sample as well. Reliability is a function of the instrument and the user. Comparable to using a scalpel, a scale may perform well in one set of hands and not in another. Clinicians should at least ponder whether their studies vary from previous studies along various dimensions (e.g., the population of interest, the study setting, the method of data collection, and interviewer background) that might threaten the reliability and validity of the measures.

Reliability

Reliability is a measure of reproducibility and is solely an empirical issue. Common types of reliability are internal, test–retest, and interrater. One may be interested in reproducibility of individual test scores across similar items in a test, of individual test scores over time, and of individual test scores by different observers. Specifically, the investigator must have repeated measures across some dimension (e.g., multiple items measuring the same construct, multiple test scores over time for the same subjects, and multiple raters scoring the same patients). Fundamentally, reliability can be expressed as follows (Carmines & Zeller, 1979; Crocker & Algina, 1986; Streiner & Norman, 1995):

$$\text{Reliability} = \frac{\text{true variance}}{\text{true variance} + \text{error variance}}$$

This reliability coefficient, a form of an intraclass correlation coefficient (ICC), is interpreted as the percentage of variance in a measure that results from true patient (or respondent) variability. The ICC provides information on the "extent to which repetition of the test yields the same values under the same conditions in the same individuals" (Guyatt, Walter, & Norman, 1987, p. 172). For all reliability coefficients, a coefficient of 1 would indicate perfect reliability (i.e., no measurement error), and a coefficient of 0 represents no reliability. Since the ICC is based on analysis of variance (ANOVA) techniques, it is appropriately used only with continuous data.

A common form of *internal reliability* used with scales is Chronbach's alpha coefficient, which is a derivation of the ICC. (The Kuder-Richardson Formula 20 is appropriate for dichotomous data; Kuder & Richardson, 1937). This type of reliability is referred to as *internal consistency*, that is, the items in the scale are homogeneous. All variability other than error variance and item variance is treated as fixed, since multiple observations occur due to the items in the scale rather than multiple observers. The formula for Chronbach's alpha coefficient is as follows (Chronbach, 1951):

$$\alpha = \frac{n}{n-1} \left[1 - \frac{\sum \sigma_i^2}{\sigma_T^2} \right]$$

n = the number of items in the scale
σ_i = the standard deviation of each scale item
σ_T = the standard deviation of the total scale score

High values of alpha occur when the items comprising the total scale score are highly correlated. If the correlation between all possible pairs of items in the scale were zero, the scale would have zero reliability. High levels of the alpha coefficient should be taken with a grain of salt, since they are sensitive to the number of items in the scale. By increasing the number of items in a scale, internal consistency seems to be increasing, but this may not actually be the case. It is possible that some of these scale items may be redundant or poor indicators of the characteristic of interest. An adequate level of α for scales used to compare groups is .70 to .80 (Nunnally & Bernstein, 1994). Examining internal consistency using the item-total correlation is also a popular method. Items in a scale that do not correlate highly with the total score minus that item are not desirable.

Another form of reliability is *test–retest reliability*. The same test is given to the same individuals after a period of time elapses. The correlation between the scores from each test is considered the reliability of the measure. Reliability may be overestimated as a result of memory if the time interval between the tests is too short, or reliability may be underestimated if the time interval is too long and real changes within respondents occur. It is not possible to separate this form of reliability from the stability of the measure (Pedhazur & Schmelkin, 1991). Thus, a "Catch 22" exists when dealing with stability of measurement and outcomes research since researchers are inherently measuring change. Thus, "We cannot be certain about the degree that functional status fluctuates without reliable measurements, and we cannot readily test the measures for reliability without assuming some stability over time in the characteristic measured" (Kane and Kane, 1981).

Kappa (κ) is a commonly used statistic to assess *interrater* agreement in situations with dichotomous outcomes (i.e., nominal scales) such as presence or absence of a condition when more than one observer/rater is used. The kappa moves beyond a measure of simple agreement by taking into account the proportion of responses that are expected by chance:

$$\kappa = \frac{P_o - P_e}{1 - P_e}$$

P_o is the observed proportion of agreement (the addition of the diagonal elements of a 2×2 table divided by the total number of responses). P_e is the expected agreement between the two raters for the two outcomes given the marginal distributions of a 2×2 table. An hypothetical example is shown in Table 9–2. The expected agreement for presence of depression is calculated as $(80 \times 100)/200 = 40$, and the expected agreement for absence of the condition is calculated as $(120 \times 100)/200 = 60$. The total expected agreement (P_e) is calculated as $(40 + 60)/200 = .5$. Kappa $= .1$ since agreement is little better than what was expected by chance. The κ value is very sensitive to the marginals; if the marginals are not well balanced, κ value will be low even when agreement is high (Feinstein & Cicchetti, 1990). This measure is appropriate only for nominal data. However, attempts have been made to develop a weighted κ for use with ordinal data. The weighted κ focuses on disagreement, typically using quadratic weights calculated as the square of the amount of discrepancy from exact agreement (Streiner & Norman, 1995). Using Pearson's correlation, percentage of agreement, and chi-square are

Table 9–2 Example of Interrater Reliability

| | Rater 1 | | |
Rater 2	Presence of depression	Absence of depression	Total
Presence of depression	45	55	100
Absence of depression	35	65	100
Total	80	120	200

not recommended for assessing interrater reliability (Bartko, 1991; Streiner & Norman, 1995).

The classical test theory notion of reliability as a ratio of true variance to total variance is limiting, since it does not break down multiple sources of error. Essentially, each type of reliability coefficient discussed above yields a different estimate of reliability. For some studies with multiple potential sources of error, total variability may be seen more practically as the sum of all variability in the measure that includes both patient/respondent variability (between subject) and measurement error (within subject) and other forms of variability, such as observer, site, or training, if the investigator deems it appropriate. *Generalizability theory*, an extension of ANOVA techniques, examines all measured sources of variance simultaneously and can address all types of reliability in a single study (Crocker & Algina, 1986). This technique has not been well utilized in the health sciences literature. This is the most appropriate approach to interrater reliability.

When assessing reliability, it is important to keep in mind that it is a measure of reproducibility, not a measure of accuracy. It does not specifically deal with the issues of sensitivity and specificity. *Sensitivity* is the ability to detect those who have a disease, and *specificity* is the ability to detect those who do not. These determinations incorporate an established cut-point for the characteristic of interest and the prevalence of the characteristic in the population.

Validity

Establishing the reliability of a measure is important, but without establishing its validity, the measure is of little worth. *Validity* lies at the heart of the measurement process, since it addresses whether the scale is measuring what it was intended to measure. However, validity is difficult to establish, since it is subject to many confounding factors. For example, abstract ideas turned into scales are subject to the definitional whims of the individual clinician or investigator (i.e., naming a factor score from a factor analysis). Also, the interview situation may affect whether one measures what is intended. An interview of a nursing home resident on the topic of quality of life in the nursing home conducted in the presence of the nursing home administrator may produce invalid results. Results could also be affected if the interview was conducted by telephone or with a proxy rather than face to face with the resident. Given all the possibilities of bias, validity becomes a matter of degree since a perfectly valid indicator is not achievable.

In practice, validity is a process of hypothesis testing that moves beyond operational definitions to demonstrate relationships between the measure of interest and other measures or observable physical properties. According to Streiner and Norman, "validating a scale is really a process whereby we determine the degree of confidence we can place on inferences we make about people based on their scores from that scale" (1995, p. 146). Although all types of validity boil down to the same thing, a whole body of literature exists on the different types and complexities of validity. Validity is a unitary concept, and types of validity are merely a useful tool for discussion. One does not get three chances to establish validity (Guion, 1980). Generally, the three main types of validity discussed are criterion-related validity, content validity, and construct validity. The investigator is responsible for determining the approach to assessing validity that best suits the construct of interest.

1. *Criterion-related validity* is assessed by correlating the measure of interest with a gold standard or an already well established measure of the characteristic (the criterion). This correlation can be assessed concurrently to establish concurrent validity, or it can be assessed in the future to establish predictive validity. An example of predictive validity would be the development and use of a new section on the medical school entrance exam to predict an individual's likelihood of pursuing primary care. One would not be able to know how well the section did at predicting the percentage of new primary care doctors until the class of medical school students graduated. Using the results of this exam section for admission or other type of decision prior to graduation will bias the correlation. The main problem with this type of validity is that the more abstract the concept is, the less likely it will be to find a criterion for assessing a measure of it. In clinical practice, screening tests often are validated using a more comprehensive diagnosis as a criterion score.

2. *Content validity* assesses the degree to which the items in the measure cover the domain of interest. For example, how well does a specific ADL scale represent the entire range of disability? The more representative the sample of disability, the more valid one's inferences will be. If the scale does not take into account difficulty of dressing and bathing, one may obtain an inaccurate picture of the extent of an individual's ability to function independently. The

main problem with content validity is that, in the health sciences, it is generally impossible to sample all of the domain due to the fuzziness of many of the concepts. For many measures, content validity reduces to a form of *face validity*, which is the judgment by the medical or research community that the measure really measures the construct and perhaps even the judgment of the respondents that the questions in the measure make sense.

3. *Construct validity* refers to the validity of measures of unobservable constructs. Since the measures cannot be observed and have no agreed-upon criteria or content, construct validity is an exercise in hypothesis testing, where the construct of interest is one of the variables. Investigators are interested in whether the scores on the measure of the construct reflect their hypotheses about patient behavior. Some common methods of establishing construct validity follow.

First, one can examine group differences on the measure. If one expects two groups to differ in a predicted manner on a measure, this can be directly tested. Often investigators administer the scale to a group of individuals known to have the characteristic of interest and a group known not to have the characteristic. It is expected that the group known to have the characteristic will score higher on the measure than the other group. However, this method neglects the fact that, in practice, the scale will need to discriminate among individuals in the middle range of the trait (Streiner & Norman, 1995).

Second, correlational studies help determine convergent and discriminant validity. If two scales both are supposed to measure functional disability (preferably using two different methods), they should be highly correlated; this is *convergent validity*. Two scales measuring different constructs, such as functional disability and mental health, should not be highly correlated; this is *discriminant validity*.

Third, Campbell and Fiske (1959) proposed a model for interpreting traits across methods. The multitrait, multimethod matrix presents all of the intercorrelations resulting when each of several traits is measured by each of several methods. This method is based on the concept that reliability is the agreement between two efforts to measure the same trait through maximally similar methods. Validity is represented in the agreement between two attempts to measure the same trait using maximally different methods. See Campbell and Fiske (1959) for a complete description.

Fourth, *confirmatory factor analysis* is used to determine whether or not the data are consistent with an underlying theoretical model, that is, whether there is in fact a unique construct. This process of validation deals with the internal structure of the construct. Pedhazur and Schmelkin, p. 66 (1991) describe factor analysis as "a family of analytic techniques designed to identify factors, or dimensions, that underlie the relations among a set of observed variables . . . the observed variables are the indicators (measures, items) presumed to reflect the construct (i.e., the factor)."

Construct validity is an ongoing process. Ideally, construct validation requires a pattern of consistent findings involving different investigators using different theoretical structures across a number of different studies (Carmines & Zeller, 1979). Unfortunately, the house of cards investigators build trying to validate a measure can be easily toppled by a few inconsistent findings.

HOW CAN A MEASURE'S SENSITIVITY TO CHANGE BE ASSESSED?

A goal of the medical community is to produce positive change in patient health status through appropriate treatment of disease. A goal of outcomes research is to assess the effectiveness of medical treatment. Necessarily, many outcome measures are expected to be able to measure change over time in order to assess effectiveness. Besides reliability and validity, researchers argue that measures used to assess treatment effects must be responsive to changes in patient health status over time (Guyatt et al., 1987, 1989; Kirshner & Guyatt, 1985). This property is often called *responsiveness* or *sensitivity to change* in the literature. One can have reliable instruments that are not responsive and responsive instruments that are not reliable. For example, a repeated measure may give the same results every time, but it is unresponsive if it does not detect improvements in functioning that are known to have occurred. Good reliability only demonstrates that the measure adequately discriminates between individuals at a point in time. If the goal of measurement is to detect change due to treatment through group differences, a measure that reflects the responsiveness of the scale to change is needed.

Assessing the effects of medical interventions often involves the use of change scores (i.e., mean change in the outcome variable over time). However, using the reliability of the change score as a measure of responsiveness is inappropriate. A uniform response to treatment would result in a change-score reliability coefficient of zero, since the variance of the change-score is zero if all patients improve an equal amount (Streiner & Norman, 1995). To assess responsiveness, Guyatt et al. (1987) suggest creating a ratio of the clinically important difference (if available) to the variability of scores within stable patients. If the clinically important difference is unavailable, the mean change score is used. Others correlate change scores on the scale to change scores of physiologic measures (Meenan et al., 1984) or use receiver operating characteristic (ROC) curves to determine the ability of the scale to detect a clinically important change compared to some external criterion (Deyo & Centor, 1986). An ROC curve is a graph with sensitivity on the Y-axis and specificity on the X-axis. The ROC curve portrays the trade-offs involved for specificity and sensitivity of various thresholds of a given measure.

Using change scores for responsiveness seems to be an intuitive choice, since clinicians are concerned about health status before and after a medical intervention. Also, investigators argue that besides addressing responsiveness, change scores are necessary to correct for baseline differences between the experimental and control group, particularly in nonrandomized trials. However, several researchers caution the use of change scores. Norman (1989) argues that none of these methods establishes the statistical connection between reliability and responsiveness (expressed as a ratio of variances) that has been shown to exist. (See earlier reliability section.) Change scores should not be used unless the variance between subjects exceeds the error variance within subjects or more practically, unless the reliability of the measure exceeds .5 (Norman, 1989). Responsiveness can be viewed as follows (Norman, 1989; Streiner & Norman, 1995):

$$\textbf{Responsiveness} = \frac{\text{variance due to change}}{\text{variance due to change} + \text{error variance}}$$

A unitless measure of responsiveness results that expresses the proportion of variance in the change score due to true change resulting from the treatment. Nunnally further cautions that "the major problem in working directly with the change score is that they are ridden with a regression effect" (i.e., regression to the mean; 1975, p. 112). Patients who were above the mean prior to treatment tend to have negative change scores (do worse) after treatment, and patients who scored below the mean prior to treatment tend to have positive change scores (do better) due to random variation. To address this phenomenon, residualized change scores (i.e., difference between actual post test score and post test score predicted by a regression equation) are suggested for assessing individual change and analysis of covariance techniques for overall treatment effects (Chronbach & Furby, 1970; Streiner & Norman, 1995). Unfortunately, neither of these methods handle error effectively or perform well in quasiexperimental designs (Nunnally, 1975).

HOW ARE CHANGES IN HEALTH STATUS MEASURES INTERPRETED?

A reliable, valid, and responsive health status measure still has one final hurdle before it can achieve widespread use in the clinical community. Changes in health status measures must be understood by clinicians (i.e., what constitutes a meaningful or clinically significant change on the measure). Treatments may be statistically significant without being clinically significant. This phenomenon occurs more frequently in large samples, since statistical significance can be achieved with very small differences between the treatment and control group. For example, a group of stroke patients without the use of an arm enroll in a trial to examine various forms of physical therapy. One of those therapies electrically stimulates and strengthens an individual's muscles in the arm. Over time, a statistically significant improvement in the strength of that arm muscle can be detected between the treatment ($n = 5,000$) and control ($n = 5,000$) groups. However, most of the patients do not have any associated improvement in the ability to use the arm in daily living.

Attempts at interpretation have been either distribution based or anchor based (Deyo & Patrick, 1995). *Distribution-based interpretation* typically involves the *effect size*, which is the mean change in a variable divided by the standard deviation of that variable (Cohen, 1977). Kazis, Anderson, and Meenan (1989) believe that translating changes in health status into a standard unit of measurement and using general–effect-size thresholds provide a clearer understanding of clinical significance. General–effect-size thresholds are: .2 is a small effect, .5 is a moderate effect, and .8 is a large effect (Cohen, 1977). Unfortunately, for some interventions a .2 may be clinically significant, and a .8 may not be clinically significant in others. For comparison of health status scores across instruments, some argue that the denominator of the effect size should be the standard deviation of the change in scores (Katz et al., 1992).

Anchor-based interpretations tie the health status measure to external measures or events. Changes in score on quality of life instruments have been calibrated to patient global ratings of change with the effect that a .5 change on a 7-point Likert scale represented clinical significance (Jaeschke, Singer, & Guyatt, 1989). Changes in mental health scores for a population of schizophrenic patients are related to the probability of subsequent major life events, such as psychiatric hospitalization, arrest, victimization, and suicide attempt (Harman et al., in process). From a policy perspective, differences in mental health scores resulted in differential use of outpatient mental health services; individuals in the lowest third of scores (sickest) had three times the average expenditures as those in the highest third (Ware et al., 1984). For other examples of anchoring health status, see Deyo and Patrick, 1995.

HOW DO MULTIPLE- VERSUS SINGLE-ITEM MEASURES COMPARE?

Three good reasons to choose multiple-item scales over single questions are improved reliability, scope, and precision (Haley, McHorney, & Ware, 1994; Nunnally & Bernstein, 1994; Spector, 1992). Single-item scales are not as reliable as multiple-item scales, since multiple-item scales average out measurement error in a construct when they are summed to obtain a total score. Generally, individual items have considerable measurement error, but it is not typically assessed. Second, in many clinical instances, a single item is inadequate to capture the complexity of a construct (e.g., quality of life, depression). Finally, multiple-item scales make it possible to discriminate more finely between the degrees of an attribute. Categorical response sets allow more discrimination than a simple yes/no question. For example, asking whether individuals can dress independently, can dress with limited help from assistive devices or by taking excessive time, can dress with help from another person, or is unable to dress provides more information on the level of disability than simply asking whether the individual dresses without assistance. Several aggregated, multiple-category questions measuring a single construct provide many times the precision.

WHAT ARE THE SHORTCOMINGS OF TRADITIONAL MULTIPLE-ITEM SCALES?

Multiple-item scales are preferable to single variables for complex constructs, but several shortcomings of traditional test theory and scale construction make these scales less than perfect (Crocker & Algina, 1986; Hambleton & Swaminathan, 1985; Streiner & Norman, 1995). First, on such scales, it is not possible to determine how people with different levels of a characteristic perform on a given item of the scale. Each scale item is assumed to tap the underlying characteristic identically. Second, scales are not generally test-free or sample-free. Individuals that complete different items on a scale cannot be compared (test-free) nor can scales generally be used in different groups without reestablishing the psychometric properties (e.g., reliability and validity) of the scale (scale-free).

In theory, a scale constructed according to item response theory (IRT) will be sample- and test-free. The scale will be reproducible across diverse groups and over repeated tests. Psychometric properties will not need to be reestablished. Individuals completing different items on the scale can easily be scored and compared. For example, scores of impaired individuals completing the easiest 10 items on the scale could be compared to the scores of unimpaired individuals completing the most difficult 7 items. This method of scaling is an extension of Guttman scaling. Thus, a hierarchical structure is assumed. Also, the items in the scale can only measure a single underlying trait (*unidimensionality*), and the probability of answering Item J positively is not related to the probability of answering Item K positively (*local independence*). Local independence would be unmet if Item K depended on Item J or earlier items. Health-related scale applications of IRT are limited but gaining popularity (Avlund, Kreiner, & Schultz-Larson, 1993; Fisher & William, 1993; Haley et al., 1994).

Rather than the deterministic method of Guttman scaling, which assumes no error, IRT is based on the probability of responding positively to a scale item based on the amount of the underlying trait that an individual possesses. The more of a trait an individual has, the more likely he or she will respond positively to the scale item. Specifically, IRT is based on the "probability that a randomly chosen member of a homogeneous group will respond correctly to an item" (Crocker & Algina, 1986, p. 341). Item characteristic curves are plots of the relationship between the person's performance on any item and the underlying trait (Streiner & Norman, 1995). (See Figure 9–2.) The curves are S-shaped and based on the logistic curve.

Three logistic IRT models are in use and vary in their levels of complexity. The models vary on three parameters: (a) discrimination or steepness of slope, (b) difficulty or location along the trait continuum, and (c) guessing or where the bottom of the item characteristic curve flattens (Streiner & Norman, 1995). In the one-parameter model, the item characteristic curves represent the proportion of individuals responding positively as a function of the latent trait and the difficulty of the item. The one-parameter model is equivalent to the Rasch model. In the two-parameter model, the item characteristic curves represent the proportion of individuals responding positively to an item as a function of the latent trait, the difficulty of the item, and the discrimination of the item. In the three parameter model, the item characteristic curves represent the proportion of individuals responding positively as a function of the latent trait, the difficulty of the item, the discrimination of the item, and guessing on the item. Following is the formula for the probability (P_i) that a randomly chosen member of a homogeneous group will respond correctly to an item:

$$Pi(v) = \frac{e^k}{1 + e^k}$$

one-parameter model: $k = a\,(\Theta - b_i)$
two-parameter model: $k = a_i\,(\Theta - b_i)$
three-parameter model: $k = a_i\,(\Theta - b_i)$

$$P_i\,(\Theta) = c_i + \frac{(1 - c_i)\,e^k}{1 + e^k}$$

Θ = amount of the latent trait
a = discrimination: the ability of an item to discriminate between different levels of the trait (the slope of the item characteristic curve)
b = difficulty: the greater the difficulty, the more latent trait the respondent must have to score positively on the scale (location of the item characteristic curve on the trait (x) axis)
c = pseudo-guessing parameter: accounts for guessing in people with low levels of the trait (item characteristic curve does not approach zero)

In Figure 9–2, the scale item represented by item characteristic curve z is more difficult than the scale item for item characteristic curve x. One must have more of the trait to respond positively to the scale item for item characteristic curve z.

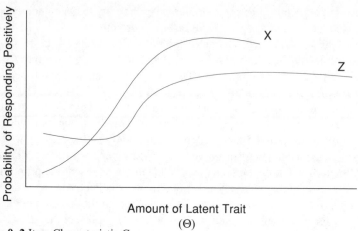

Figure 9–2 Item Characteristic Curves

The scale item for item characteristic curve x discriminates better (steeper slope) than the item for item characteristic curve z. Item characteristic curve z shows that the probability of responding positively to the item is never less than 10% due to guessing by individuals with low levels of the trait.

Choosing the appropriate model depends on whether guessing could be a problem and whether items in the scale are believed to tap levels of the underlying trait differentially. The less complex the model, the more accurate and easier it is to estimate. The investigator must consider the effects on the results when all the assumptions of IRT are not met (Crocker & Algina, 1986). Moreover, classical reliability measures can be translated for use with IRT applications, but validity is still a concern. Latent traits are not the same thing as constructs; IRT does not provide a guarantee that items are measuring what they were intended to measure (Crocker & Algina, 1986). A latent trait may be responsible for the performance of a set of items, but these items may not be tapping the construct that was intended. Goodness-of-fit measures to assess how well the model fits the data are still under development, especially for the two- and three-parameter models.

Ideally, IRT enables the creation of test-free and sample-free measurement. A scale representing a hierarchy of a trait allows people to be compared even if they chose different items on the scale or are from different subpopulations. Potential economies of scale in scale administration are possible. However, large sample sizes are generally needed to estimate these models (minimum of 200 for the one-parameter model and 1,000 for the three-parameter model) as well as specialized software (Crocker & Algina, 1986). Also, a good understanding of the trait is essential to construct items for a unidimensional scale.

WHAT ABOUT MEASUREMENT ERROR?

Poor measurement has serious implications for analysis of the data. Calculating the variance of a single variable measured with error results in an overestimate of the variance. In multiple regression analysis, one assumes that each variable is measured without error. For reasons discussed earlier, this is an unrealistic assumption. When variables are measured with error, estimation problems result (Kmenta, 1986). Random measurement error in the dependent variable (left side of the equation) yields unbiased regression coefficients, but the R squared (i.e., the total variance explained by the model) is decreased. Random measurement error in independent variables (right side of the equation) will produce biased and inconsistent regression coefficients, so these coefficients should not be used for confidence intervals and t-tests. Measurement error in only one independent variable in the regression model will affect the coefficients of variables free of error, and it will not be possible to determine the direction of the bias in the coefficients (Bollen, 1989). Alternative methods of coefficient estimation are needed in the presence of measurement error (Bollen, 1989; Kmenta, 1986).

Through the process of using a measurement model, unobservable or observed constructs are operationalized by connecting them to one or more observed measures. Unobserved latent variables are typically associated with a sizable amount of measurement error. Developing a multiple-item scale of an unobservable construct averages out the measurement error, but the psychometric properties of the scale (e.g., reliability and validity) still remain a function of the sample used in the development of the scale. Measurement error in a single-item measure is rarely addressed; it is not possible to calculate a Chronbach's alpha for this type of measure.

When using unobserved constructs in a model, *latent variable structural equation modeling* offers a potential advantage over traditional analysis techniques, such as multiple regression, since it involves both a measurement model (confirmatory factor analysis) and structural equation modeling (less restrictive regression modeling). Latent variable structural equation modeling allows the investigator to estimate accurately both direct and indirect causal relationships among the variables in the face of measurement error and causality that does not flow in a single direction; traditional regression approaches do not allow this (Joreskog & Sorbom, 1989). Multiple indicators are used to measure the latent variables in the model. For example, family socioeconomic status may be measured by four variables: parental educational attainment, types of jobs held by the parents, size of home, and family income. Using multiple indicators allows the reliabilities and validities of the variable to be estimated directly. The coefficients are unbiased since all random and nonrandom error is extracted by the measurement model. The latent variable structural equation model uses only the true variance associated with each variable to estimate the coefficients. (See Figure 9–3.)

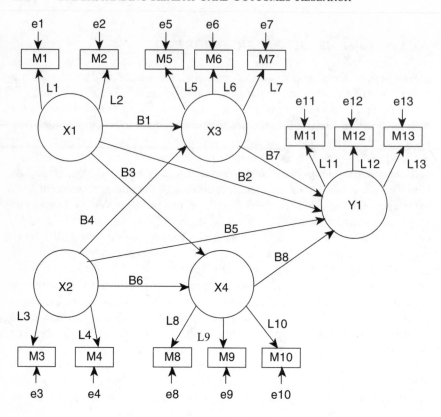

Figure 9–3 Latent Variable Structural Equation Model. The measurement model component of the figure shows multiple indicators (M) measuring each latent variable. The Ls (factor loadings) show the strength of the relationship between each indicator and the latent variable. Random measurement error (e) in the latent variables is taken into account by the measurement model. Non-random error can be taken into account by correlating the errors across indicators (e.g., e2 covaries with e5). The Bs (regression coefficients) represent the direct and indirect causal relationships between the latent variables in the model.

CONCLUSION

Measurement can involve some extremely complex elements. It is an important—but deceptive—component of the overall process of assessing outcomes. Because the issues appear to address attributes that are familiar, they seem readily accessible. In essence, measurement involves creating abstract representations for clinical realities. These conceptions are often fragile entities and must be handled with care. As statistical capacities expand, the numbers of assumptions also increase. Investigators must at least be sensitive to the potential pitfalls and willing to accept the idea that they exist even when they are not recognized by untrained eyes. In many cases, technical assistance is needed from experts who are familiar with measurement and its subtle complexities.

REFERENCES

Andresen, E.M., Patrick, D.L., Carter, W.B., & Malmgren, J.A. (1995). Comparing the performance of health status measures for older adults. *Journal of the American Geriatrics Society, 43*(9), 1,030–1,034.

Avlund, K., Kreiner, S., & Schultz-Larson, K. (1993). Construct validation and the Rasch model: Functional ability of healthy elderly people. *Scandinavian Journal of Social Medicine, 21*(4), 233–245.

Bartko, J. (1991). Measurement and reliability: Statistical thinking considerations. *Schizophrenia Bulletin, 17*(3), 483–489.

Blalock, J., & Hubert, M. (1982). *Conceptualization and measurement in the social sciences.* Beverly Hills, CA: Sage Publications.

Bollen, K.A. (1989). *Structural Equations with Latent Variables.* New York: John Wiley & Sons.

Campbell, D., & Fiske, D. (1959). Convergent and discriminant validation by the multitrait-multimethod matrix. *Psychological Bulletin, 56*, 81–105.

Carmines, E.G., & Zeller, R.A. (1979). *Reliability and validity assessment.* Beverly Hills, CA: Sage Publications.

Chronbach, L. (1951). Coefficient alpha and the internal structure of tests. *Psychometrika, 16*, 297–334.

Chronbach, L., & Furby, L. (1970). How we should measure "change"—or should we? *Psychological Bulletin, 74*, 68–80.

Cohen, J. (1977). *Statistical power analysis for the behavioral sciences.* New York: Academic Press.

Crocker, L., & Algina, J. (1986). *Introduction to classical and modern test theory.* New York: Holt, Rinehart, and Winston.

DeVellis, R.F. (1991). *Scale development: Theories and applications.* Newbury Park, CA: Sage Publications.

Deyo, R.A., & Centor, R.M. (1986). Assessing the responsiveness of functional scales to clinical change: An analogy to diagnostic test performance. *Journal of Chronic Disease, 39*(11), 897–906.

Deyo, R.A., & Patrick, D.L. (1995). The significance of treatment effects: The clinical perspective. *Medical Care, 33*(4), AS286–AS291.

Duncan, O.D. (1984). *Notes on social measurement: Historical and critical.* New York: Russell Sage Foundation.

Feinstein, A., & Cicchetti, D. (1990). High agreement but low kappa: I. The problems of two paradoxes. *Journal of Clinical Epidemiology, 43*(6), 543–549.

Finch, M., Kane, R.L., & Philp, I. (1995). Developing a new metric for ADLs. *Journal of the American Geriatrics Society, 43*(8), 877–884.

Fisher, J., & William, P. (1993). Measurement related problems in functional assessment. *The American Journal of Occupational Therapy, 47*(4), 331–338.

Guion, R.M. (1980). On trinitarian doctrines of validity. *Professional Psychology, 11*, 385–398.

Guyatt, G., Walter, S., & Norman, G. (1987). Measuring change over time: Assessing the usefulness of evaluative instruments. *Journal of Chronic Diseases, 40*(2), 171–178.

Guyatt, G.H., Deyo, R.A., Charlson, M., Levine, M.N., & Mitchell, A. (1989). Responsiveness and validity in health status measurement: A clarification. *Journal of Clinical Epidemiology, 42*(5), 403–408.

Haley, S.M., McHorney, C.A., & Ware, J.E.J. (1994). Evaluation of the MOS SF-36 physical functioning scale (PF-10): I. Unidimensionality and reproducibility of the Rasch item scale. *Journal of Clinical Epidemiology, 47*(6), 671–684.

Hambleton, R., & Swaminathan, H. (1985). *Item response theory: Principles and applications.* Boston: Kluwer Nijhoff.

Harman, J.S., Manning, W.G., Lurie, N., Liu, C.F., Popkin, M.K., & Gray, D.Z. (in process, p. 233). Interpreting clinical and policy significance in mental health services research. Unpublished manuscript.

Hoeymans, N., Feskens, E.J., van den Bos, G.A., & Kromhout, D. (1996). Measuring functional status: Cross-sectional and longitudinal associations between performance and self-report (Zutphen Elderly Study 1990–1993). *Journal of Clinical Epidemiology, 49*(10), 1,103–1,110.

Jaeschke, R., Singer, J., & Guyatt, G.H. (1989). Measurement of health status: Ascertaining the minimal clinically important difference. *Controlled Clinical Trials, 10*(4), 407–415.

Joreskog, K.G., & Sorbom, D. (1989). *LISREL 7: A guide to the program and application.* (2nd ed.). Chicago: SPSS.

Kane, R.A., & Kane, R.L. (1981). *Assessing the elderly: A practical guide to measurement.* Lexington, MA: D.C. Heath.

Kaplan, R.M. (1995). Utility assessment for estimating quality-adjusted life years. In F.A. Sloan (Ed.), *Valuing health care,* (pp. 31–60). New York: Cambridge University Press.

Katz, J.N., Larson, M.G., Phillips, C.B., Fossel, A.H., & Liang, M.H. (1992). Comparative measurement sensitivity of short and longer health status instruments. *Medical Care, 30*(10), 917–925.

Katz, S., Ford, A.B., Moskowitz, R.W., Jackson, B.A., & Jaffe, M.W. (1963). Studies of illness in the aged. The index of ADL: A standardized measure of biological and psychosocial function. *JAMA, 185,* 914–919.

Kazis, L.E., Anderson, J.J., & Meenan, R.F. (1989). Effect sizes for interpreting changes in health status. *Medical Care, 27*(Suppl. 3), S178–S189.

Kirshner, B., & Guyatt, G. (1985). A methodological framework for assessing health indices. *Journal of Chronic Disease, 27*(3), S178–S189.

Kmenta, J. (1986). *Elements of econometrics.* (2nd ed.). New York: Macmillan Publishing.

Kuder, G., & Richardson, M. (1937). The theory of the estimation of test reliability. *Psychometrika, 2,* 151–160.

Lazaridis, E.N., Rudberg, M.A., Furner, S.E., & Cassel, C.K. (1994). Do activities of daily living have a hierarchical structure? An analysis using the longitudinal study of aging. *Journal of Gerontology: Medical Sciences, 49*(2), M47–M51.

Magaziner, J., Simonsick, E., Kashner, E., & Hebel, J. (1988). Patient-proxy response comparability on measures of patient health and functional status. *Journal of Clinical Epidemiology, 41*(11), 1,065–1,074.

Maruyama, G. (in press). *Basics of structural equation modeling.* Thousand Oaks, CA: SAGE.

McDowell, I., & Newell, C. (1996). *Measuring health: A guide to rating scales and questionnaires.* New York: Oxford University Press.

McIver, J.P., & Carmines, E.G. (1981). *Unidimensional Scaling.* Newbury Park, CA: Sage Publications.

Meenan, R., Anderson, J., Kazis, L., Egger, M., Altz-Smith, M., & Samuelson, C.O., Jr. (1984). Outcome assessment in clinical trials: Evidence for the sensitivity of a health status measure. *Arthritis and Rheumatism, 27*(12), 1,344–1,352.

Norman, G.R. (1989). Issues in the use of change scores in randomized trials. *Journal of Clinical Epidemiology, 42*(11), 1,097–1,105.

Nunnally, J.C. (1975). The study of change in evaluation research: Principles concerning measurement, experimental design, and analysis. In E.L. Struening & M. Guttentag (Eds.), *Handbook of evaluation research,* (vol. 1, pp. 101–138). Beverly Hills, CA: Sage Publications.

Nunnally, J.C., & Bernstein, I.H. (1994). *Psychometric theory.* (3rd ed.). New York: McGraw-Hill.

Pedhazur, E.J., & Schmelkin, L.P. (1991). *Measurement, design, and analysis: An integrated approach.* (Student ed.). Hillsdale, NJ: Lawrence Erlbaum Associates.

Rubenstein, L., Schairer, C., Wieland, G., & Kane, R. (1984). Systematic biases in functional status of assessment of elderly adults: Effects of different data sources. *The Journal of Gerontology, 39*(6), 686–691.

Spector, P.E. (1992). *Summated rating scale construction: An introduction.* Newbury Park, CA: Sage Publications.

Stevens, S.S. (1981). Measurement. In G. Maranell (Ed.), *SCALING: A sourcebook for behavioral scientists* (2nd ed., pp. 22–41). Chicago: Aldine Publishing.

Streiner, D., & Norman, G. (1995). *Health measurement scales: A practical guide to their development and use* (2nd ed.). New York: Oxford University Press.

Torrance, G., & Feeny, D. (1989). Utilities and quality-adjusted life years. *International Journal of Technology Assessment in Health Care, 5*(4), 559–575.

Travis, S.S., & McAuley, W.J. (1990). Simple counts of the number of basic ADL dependencies for long-term care research and practice. *HSR: Health Services Research, 25*(2), 349–360.

Tversky, A., & Kahneman, D. (1981). The framing of decisions and the psychology of choice. *Science, 211,* 453–458.

Ware, J.E. Jr., Manning, W.G., Duan, N., Wells, K.B., & Newhouse, J.P. (1984). Health status and the use of outpatient mental health services. *American Psychologist, 39*(10), 1,090–1,100.

Weiss, A., Fletcher, A.E., Palmer, A.J., Nicholl, C.G., & Bulpitt, C.J. (1996). Use of surrogate respondents in studies of stroke and dementia. *Journal of Clinical Epidemiology, 49*(10), 1,187–1,194.

Young, N.L., Williams, J.I., Yoshida, K.K., Bombardier, C., & Wright, J.G. (1996). The context of measuring disability: Does it matter whether capability or performance is measured? *Journal of Clinical Epidemiology, 49*(10), 1,097–1,101.

10

Miscellaneous Observations about Outcomes Research: Practical Advice

Robert L. Kane

CHAPTER OUTLINE

- How Realistic Is the Search for Simple Measures?
- How Can Data Quality Be Improved?
- How Do Researchers Get Follow-Up Data?
- When Are Extant Data Sources Helpful?
- What Are the Basic Analytic Issues?
- What Ethical Issues Should Outcomes Researchers Keep in Mind?
- Case Example

As stressed earlier in this book, a conceptual model is the foundation of the analysis. The conceptual model should indicate which variables are thought to influence the outcomes and how. A conceptual model need not be equivalent to a theoretical model, in the sense that it does not have to draw upon some grand general theory. Rather, it can be based on one's clinical experience or even beliefs about what is going on and what factors are likely to influence the outcomes of interest. Its major role is to clarify the expected relationships. Often, drawing a model illuminates the analytic problems. Such diagrams can distinguish the primary risk factors from the intervening events (including both treatments and complications of treatment) and can make clear the temporal relationships among the variables.

The capacity to account statistically for variance has become a passion in some quarters, but it is important to appreciate that the more temporally proximal a variable is to the outcome, the more variance it will usually explain. (At the extreme, cessation of respiration predicts death very well.) However, explaining variance is not always helpful. For example, cessation of respiration will undoubtedly explain much of the variation in mortality rates, but so what?

In some cases, accounting for variation may lead to false conclusions. For example, a study of the utilization of medical care by the informal caregivers of Alzheimer's disease patients showed that they appeared to use less care than controls. The investigators had earlier identified that depression was more common among caregivers, so they controlled for this difference in their analysis to render the two groups more comparable. However, a causal model might well suggest that the development of depression was a result of caregiving and a determinant of medical care use. Controlling for such a step would dramatically dampen the effects of giving this stressful care and misstate the effects of caregiving.

The conceptual model needs to make clear not only the relationship between various antecedents and the outcomes but also the relationship among the various outcomes themselves. In some instances, the outcomes may be seen as parallel, but, in many cases, they will assume some sort of hierarchical form, where one may be expected to lead to the next. The discussion of this measurement hierarchy and its role in relating outcomes to interventions (covered in Chapter 9) is very relevant here (Spiegel et al., 1986).

In planning an outcomes study, it is important to identify in advance which outcome is the primary one, the basis on which success or failure can be ultimately judged. Many interventions can be expected to achieve a variety of results, but, in the end, one outcome must be identified as the most significant. This decision will, among other things, affect the choice of what variables to use in calculating the necessary sample size to obtain statistical power.

A priori identification of the major outcome does not preclude retrospective insight, but it should cast it in a different light. It is reasonable, even desirable, that greater understanding about the relationship between treatments and outcomes occurs after one has systematically studied the problem. There is nothing wrong with postulating new relationships or embellishing the prior models, but one must appreciate that such post hoc reasoning is not causal; it represents hypothesis formulation, not hypothesis testing. It should be conducted, but it should be recognized for what it is. One cannot generate a hypothesis to apply to data after they have been analyzed, but the insights gained from such thought can be usefully applied in planning (or recommending) the next series of studies.

HOW REALISTIC IS THE SEARCH FOR SIMPLE MEASURES?

Many clinicians (and policy makers) long for a single, simple outcome. Is there a number that can be said to summarize all the outcomes of concern, akin to the

Dow Jones average or the percentage of the gross national product spent on health care or even the infant mortality rate? Most outcomes measures are too complex. The best ones usually offer a profile of results, where a provider (or a treatment) can excel in one area and fall short in another. Just as some prefer a grade-point average as the summary of a student's academic success, others look for the profile of areas of success and failure. However, as much as some may wish it, most of life cannot be summed up in a single statistic.

Moreover, providing a complex summary measure that represents the weighted average of many outcome variables may not be illuminating either. Such indexes are not immediately understandable. They lack a frame of reference. What does it mean to have a score of "x" or to have improved by "y" points? When such scale scores are used, it is useful to provide some sort of guide that can allow the reader to translate the numerical value into something more tangible and familiar; for example, "someone with a score of 'x' cannot do the following . . . or is similar to someone who is in . . . condition." (The importance of anchoring such measures in the context of life events was discussed more thoroughly in Chapter 9.)

HOW CAN DATA QUALITY BE IMPROVED?

The bane of many clinical studies is data quality. There is a basic bias that real data come from clinicians and that patient reports cannot be trusted. This bias needs to be attacked on two grounds.

1. Patient perceptions can provide very useful information. They may not be technically accurate in areas that require clinical expertise, but they may be the most valid sources for information about how they feel and how disease affects them. Filtering such information through a clinician does not always improve the noise-to-signal ratio.
2. Clinician reports are not universally useful or accurate. Often, elaborate systems are devised to review medical records reliably. Record abstractors are trained and monitored closely to ensure comparable work. However, the quality of most medical records leaves much to be desired. Not only is information recorded in incomplete ways, it is impossible to infer what an omission means. Does the lack of a comment on a physical finding or a symptom imply that nothing of interest was found or nothing was looked for? What does it mean when a record says a body system was "within normal limits"? What type of examination was actually done? What does "no history of 'x' " mean? What questions were asked? Few clinicians systematically record all the pertinent information needed to adjust for risk factors, nor do they provide complete data on which to establish outcomes.

For many variables, especially those that require judgment or interpretation, clinicians are the best source of information, even when their interrater (and perhaps even their intertemporal) reliability has not been established. Getting useful data from clinicians often means setting up some type of prospective data collection apparatus. Some means of querying the clinicians is needed to be sure that they make the complete set of observations sought and record the information consistently.

Clinicians do not generally respond well to such demands for structured information collection. Many have a strong aversion to forms, which they deprecate as some type of "cookbook medicine." In order to gain their cooperation, it is often necessary to involve them proactively in designing the data collection forms or at least identifying the relevant material to be included.

This proactive strategy is especially important in the context of quality improvement projects. Although purists will worry (justifiably) that such active involvement will bias clinician behavior, such a bias is precisely what quality improvement seeks. Those being judged are more likely to accept the results of the outcomes analysis if they have had some role in developing the criteria and the way the data are collected.

In some cases, the bias toward clinician-generated information may be misplaced. Clinicians serve as mere conduits; the data can be better collected directly from patients, who may provide more and better information without the clinician filter. For example, data on patient functioning are usually better collected directly from the patients (or their proxies). Even information on key symptoms can often be obtained more easily and better directly from patients. In some cases, office (or hospital) personnel can be trained (and induced) to collect questionnaires (or even conduct short interviews) with patients when they present themselves for care.

HOW DO RESEARCHERS GET FOLLOW-UP DATA?

While it is at least theoretically possible to structure baseline and risk factor data collection into ordinary clinical activities, obtaining follow-up information is more complicated. Even if clinicians were cooperative, problems would arise. Patients are not usually seen for follow-up appointments on a consistent schedule. Some patients are lost to follow-up. Because biased data can be very dangerous, some form of systematic data collection that does not rely on patients returning to the clinic or hospital is in order. Although such a step adds cost and represents an added dimension, its value in providing adequate unbiased coverage justifies the expense.

Follow-up data can be collected by various means. The most expensive is in-person interviews. Such a step is generally not required unless the patients are especially unreachable (e.g., nursing home patients) or data must be physically collected (e.g., blood samples, blood pressure, weight). Most times, the data can be reduced to patient reports of symptoms and behaviors, which can be collected by either mailed questionnaires or telephone interviews. The choice of which approach to use is based on money and expected compliance. Often, a mixed approach will be needed, with nonrespondents to the mailed survey contacted by telephone or even visited.

Response rates are very important. The basic concern is about response bias (where those who respond are systematically different from those who do not). In some cases, the source of the bias is obvious (e.g., those returning for follow-up care). In most cases, the reasons for nonresponse are not evident, even when interviewers ask why the patient refused to participate. The best way to avoid such a bias is to go all out to collect data on all subjects who are eligible. Inevitably, the last group to be reached will require the majority of the overall follow-up effort.

Those not familiar with research methods sometimes confuse large numbers of respondents with adequate response rates. Whereas sample size is important in determining the statistical power of an analysis, large numbers of respondents cannot compensate for poor response rates. It is usually better to use the available resources to ensure that one collects a high proportion of those targeted than just a lot of cases. A high response rate from a smaller sample is by far preferable to a larger but more incomplete sample.

In some instances, patients may not be able to respond because they are too sick or cognitively compromised. Proxy respondents can be used to obtain information, but they should be employed with caution. Often, family members will try to protect patients from such contacts, even when the patients can and want to participate. In some cases, those responsible for the patient may not want the patient to participate or may view the data collection activity as another nuisance. For example, nursing homes may find it inconvenient to get patients to a telephone to answer questions. Persistence and creativity will be needed to counter these ploys.

In some cases, proxies are inevitable. Care and common sense should be used in deciding when a proxy can accurately represent the patient. At least two criteria should apply:

1. The proxy should have recent and adequate exposure to the patient to be able to report on his or her status (e.g., family members listed as the responsible party in a hospital or nursing home may not have visited frequently enough to know what is really happening).
2. The domains proxies can address should make sense; for example, it is unrealistic to expect a proxy to report on a patient's degree of pain or the patient's state of mind.

The timing of follow-ups is important. Particularly when treatment may extend over long periods (e.g., outpatient therapy), the effects of dating follow-ups from the beginning or the end of treatment can make a huge difference. If follow-up is dated from the beginning of the treatment, and some patients remain in treatment substantially longer than others, the differences in outcomes may be attributable to the time between the end of treatment and the follow-up. Thus, it is usually safer to date follow-up from the end of treatment. However, even this precaution will not eliminate the need to pay careful attention to the duration of the treatment. As noted in Chapter 5, duration and intensity are important attributes of treatment that must be considered in the analysis of its effects.

Duration of treatment can thus have several effects. It can mask the effects of the natural course of a disease. If the disease in question has a natural history independent of treatment, a longer duration of treatment may simply allow the problem to run its course. Remaining in prolonged treatment may reflect patients' motivation and influence their recovery. If those who become discouraged drop out of treatment, it is hard to separate the effects of less treatment from inherent characteristics of the patients. Because those who drop out may also be harder to contact at follow-up, there may be a selective attrition bias.

WHEN ARE EXTANT DATA SOURCES HELPFUL?

In some cases, outcomes information can make use of extant secondary data sources. For example, Medicare records can be used to trace when a person is rehospitalized or when a given operation is revised. Using secondary data sources, especially administrative databases, can be limiting and challenging. It is no coincidence that the most common outcomes addressed are death and rehospitalization. They are the two items that most administrative databases can yield. In some circumstances, such follow-up data can provide useful adjunctive information. For example, a study of hip replacement may address short-term benefits in terms of pain and mobility, but it may also be useful to see how long the prostheses lasted.

It is important to distinguish studies that rely exclusively on secondary data and those used in conjunction with primary data. The former face problems of limited information, especially when it comes to adjusting for risk factors, most of which cannot be found in administrative data sets. While outcomes studies derived from administrative data can relatively inexpensively compare the results of large, heterogeneous groups of providers, they are often harshly criticized as being unfair and biased. For example, when Medicare data were used to compare the mortality rates among hospitals serving Medicare patients, the results were actively challenged on the grounds that they did not adequately control for differences in case mix among the hospitals (Greenfield et al., 1988; Jencks et al., 1988; Kahn et al., 1988).

WHAT ARE THE BASIC ANALYTIC ISSUES?

Although data analysis is an integral component of a successful outcomes system, this is not the place to offer a course on the topic. Many good texts and commentaries are available. Nonetheless, we do want to offer a few basic suggestions. The first and most important is to recognize the complexities of this area and to get the necessary assistance. Outcomes analysis can often be a subtle process. The statistical pitfalls are numerous.

An important step in designing an analytic strategy is to link each hypothesis or research question with a specific analysis. This translation needs to be done in considerable detail. The concepts alluded to in the hypothesis need to be translated into specific variables and the type of analysis specified. It is often helpful to create dummy tables that show just how the results will be displayed. Going through the exercise of designing those tables can help investigators (especially neophytes) clarify just how they will organize their data and what form each variable will take.

Most analyses involving outcomes will eventually use some type of multivariate analysis, which will likely fall into one or another type of regression model. Many regression models provide two types of information: the amount of variance explained (R^2) and the relationship of each independent variable to the dependent variable (*regression coefficient*). These two factors may not be related. It is possible to explain a substantial amount of the variance without a single significant coefficient, and significant variables need not contribute much to explaining the overall variance. Each item connotes something different. It is important to decide which piece of information is most salient. The explained variance can be thought of as comparable to, in epidemiological terms, absolute risk. The *absolute risk* reflects how much added risk for developing a condition a given factor poses. The individual variable coefficients are comparable to *relative risk*: how does the risk of developing the condition with the factor compare to without it? In rare events, one may encounter a high relative risk but a small absolute risk. Likewise, with outcomes, the goal may be to identify factors that influence outcomes, even if they do not explain much of the overall risk of the outcome occurring.[1]

In one respect, treatment can be viewed as one of a series of risk factors[2] that affect the outcomes of care. In most instances, the goal of the analysis is to separate the effect of treatment from the effects of the other risk factors. It is also possible, however, to use outcomes analyses to examine directly the effect of other risk factors.

In some cases, one may want to see how a risk factor performs after the effects of other factors have been controlled (i.e., What is the specific contribution of a given factor?). In other situations, the effect of other factors may be thought to have an effect on the factor of interest (i.e., there is an interaction). For example, hospital length of stay may be influenced by whether a patient is discharged to a nursing home and whether that person is covered by Medicaid. One could examine the individual contributions of each variable in a regression model. However, the effect of a nursing home discharge might be modified by the patient's Medicaid status. To test this possibility, one could look at the effect of the interaction of these two variables on the dependent variable, or one could form two subgroups (those on Medicaid and those not) and compare the effects of nursing home discharge on each.

Different types of variables will require different types of analyses. The differences may be based on the assumptions about the normality of the distribution of the variables (i.e., is the curve bell-shaped?). In general, there are two classes of analyses (parametric and nonparametric). The former are appropriately used when the dependent variable is assumed to be normally distributed. In some cases, it is possible to transform the dependent variable into a normal distribution to make such analyses more feasible. Some variables have unusual distributions. Variables like health care cost and utilization data may show a large peak near zero use and a thin, long tail of high users. That is, there may be a large number of cases in which there is no event during the observation period; many people use few, if any, services in a given year. For example, approximately 20% of Medicare enrollees will use no services in a given year. Using regular regression techniques will result in biased coefficients. Special analytic techniques have been developed to handle such cases. Categorical dependent variables (including dichotomous or polytomous) variables require different analytic techniques, usually termed *nonparametric*. Special regression techniques (e.g., logistic regression) that avoid the problem of biased coefficients are available for these circumstances.

A note of caution is in order. Care should be used in interpreting the results of regression analyses. A variety of problems can haunt such efforts, including use of too many variables for the number of observations, colinearity among the variables, endogeneity (i.e., reciprocal relationships among the dependent and independent variables), and unusual distributions that bias the coefficients or render them uninterpretable. Statistical assistance is invaluable, both when designing a study and in interpreting the results.

WHAT ETHICAL ISSUES SHOULD OUTCOMES RESEARCHERS KEEP IN MIND?

Outcomes investigators may encounter some ethical issues. For example, there is still debate about how much informed consent must be obtained from patients. In general, when an outcomes project is done as part of an ongoing quality of care process that is incorporated into a medical care system's regular activities, no special permission is required. It is assumed that the patient who initially agreed to be treated accepts the outcomes work as part of that treatment. However, if outside agencies are used to collect the data, or if it is used for more scientific purposes (or any purpose beyond direct quality improvement for the clinicians involved), then the patients must first give their permission to be interviewed or even to have their records examined.

Confidentiality is an important ethical consideration. Some institutional review boards (which must adjudicate the ethical aspects of a study) will not even permit an outside research agency to contact patients directly to request their permission to participate in a study. Simply releasing their names is seen as a breach of confidentiality. Instead, the patients' physicians must first seek their permission to be contacted. Such a step rigorously enforced can put an end to outcomes research. Few care providers have the resources to persist in following up the substantial numbers of patients who simply fail to respond to an invitation to participate. Although it would be wrong to coerce a patient into participating, it is also dangerous to eliminate from a study those who simply fail to indicate whether or not they are willing to participate. Somehow, the investigators need to be deputized to act in the physicians' stead if the study is to be conducted.

Both patients and providers need to be clear about how the material around an outcomes study will be used. When anonymity is promised, it must be complete. Under such cases, the results about a given patient cannot be shared with that patient's doctors. On the other hand, some patients may want the information shared; they should be given an opportunity to indicate such a preference. In general, outcomes information is obtained under the promise that it will be used only in aggregate form and no identifiers will be attached.

Providers also need to know in advance when they will be identified with the results. In some cases, the outcomes information may be useful to consumers in making informed choices. Anonymity would be disadvantageous. However, providers may be rightfully concerned that adequate case-mix adjustments have been made before data are released. On the other hand, failure to release identifying information can be viewed with suspicion, as if the providers had something to hide. Careful prior arrangements need to be established about how and when data will be released.

CASE EXAMPLE

Perhaps the best way to illustrate the various issues around conducting an outcomes study is to offer an example.[3] A good one is the case of a study done with a large number of Minnesota hospitals to assess the outcomes of elective chole-cystectomy (Kane et al., 1995). The study was sponsored by a consortium of hospital and medical associations at the state and county levels. The group originally had organized to develop guidelines or protocols for care management under the assumption that it was preferable to develop one's own than to use someone else's. In the course of the guidelines work, questions were raised about the quality of the database available on which to base determinations of appropriate care. It was decided that the study should be expanded to include the collection of outcomes. A study design was developed to identify the potential risk factors that should be considered in assessing the effect of treatment on the outcomes of cholecystectomy. Table 10–1 summarizes the major categories of variables used in this study according to the classification scheme used in this book.

In this case, the treatment variable of interest was initially the surgeon and the hospital where the operation was performed. The question posed was not whether performing a cholecystectomy was better than using some sort of medical treatment or even watchful waiting. Rather, the question was this: did the operation performed by one person lead to better outcomes than if done by another, and which characteristics of a case predicted better outcomes? Just as the study was being designed, a new approach to cholecystectomy was introduced: laparoscopic surgery. The study was quickly amended to include a comparison of the results of the two approaches: conventional open surgery versus laparoscopic surgery.

Clinical teams worked with outcomes researchers to establish the conceptual model. Literature reviews and meetings with clinicians were used to identify the potential risk factors that could influence the outcomes. The outcomes themselves were derived from several sources. Condition-specific measures included symptoms that were associated with indications for performing the procedure (e.g., pain, nausea). In effect, the appropriateness criteria were adapted as outcome measures under the assumption that the main purpose of the treatment was to alleviate the factors that suggested a need for care in the first place. In addition, pertinent generic measures of quality of life (e.g., ability to perform daily activities and self-rating of health status) were added. These were reviewed to ensure

Table 10–1 Variables Used in Cholecystectomy Study

Outcomes	Risk Adjustment	Treatment
Concordance with classic cholecystitis pain	Severity measures (duration, X-ray)	Open v. laparoscopic
Symptom score	Comorbidity (Charlson scale)	Hospital
Functional status	Demographics (age, gender)	Surgeon
Satisfaction (3 factors)	Prior history	

that the clinicians believed that good care would actually influence these measures.

A series of risk factors was established based on such aspects as severity and duration of the problem. Certain physiological and laboratory tests were used as criteria. After a preliminary review of some sample charts, it became quickly evident that much of the information deemed pertinent would not be available from the hospital record. The nursing departments from each of the participating hospitals were contacted to see if they would be willing to implement a special data collection activity at the time of admission. The data collected at baseline would include both specific symptom information and more generic measures; it would also be an opportunity to obtain informed consent to be contacted subsequently to ascertain follow-up status. Although the nursing staffs proved willing to undertake this added work (some were sold on the basis that this study would prove an opportunity to demonstrate the value of good nursing care as well), logistical problems did occur. As same-day surgery increased, it proved harder to obtain the baseline data: patients were not available in advance.

The follow-up data were collected by a special survey research unit. The primary data collection mode was by mail, but telephone follow-ups were used if responses were not received within the time frames allocated. This sort of follow-up plan required that patients' names and addresses be known; special procedures were used to keep the records confidential. All completed follow-ups were coded with a specific code number linked to an index. All subsequent analyses were done with only that code number. The linking of the several components of data (the baseline interviews, the follow-up questionnaires, and the medical record abstracts) was done by a small team that was part of the sponsoring organization. Careful monitoring was required to ensure that the 6-month follow-ups were collected within the time window. As soon as cases were enrolled and baseline data collected, a file was opened and the case tracked.

The medical records of each case were reviewed using a specially designed abstraction form. Interrater reliability was checked and monitored to be sure that the same information was interpreted consistently. The results of this step were combined with the baseline and follow-up data to create a single analytic file. This file had no identifiers for patients, surgeons, or hospitals. Instead, code numbers were substituted for each.

The analysis used regression models to examine the effects of the potential risk factors on the various outcomes of interest. When potential risk factors were shown to play an active role, they were retained in the models when the independent variables of major interest were introduced. The effects of laparoscopic surgery were examined by both using a dummy variable to represent the type of surgery and examining the outcomes separately for those undergoing laparoscopic and open cholecystectomies.

CONCLUSION

Outcomes research has the potential to add considerably to the empirical basis of medical practice. It will never be feasible to base all (or even a large proportion) of medical care on randomized clinical trials. On the other hand, it is irrational to assume that simply intuitively assembling the lessons of clinical experience serves as an adequate basis for scientific practice. The immediate response to the recognition of substantial variation in practice has been the institution of guidelines based largely on professional judgments about what constitutes good care. The next step is to amass the empirical database needed by those looking for a more scientific basis to establish guidelines.

Careful observations developed as part of well-designed studies will go a long way toward providing the insights needed. Researchers may never be able to say with absolute certainty that a given treatment works in a given situation, but they will have come a lot closer to making informed statements. Simply collecting data is not the answer. Studies must be carefully designed. Conceptual models must be created that combine the best of clinical and social science insights. These models should form the basis for deciding what information is to be collected and how it will be analyzed. The technology of outcomes research has come a long way in the last decades and promises to go much further. Sophisticated analytic and measurement methods are available. Like any other powerful tools, they must be handled carefully by persons skilled in their use. The best outcomes research is likely to come from partnerships of technically proficient analysts and clinicians, each of whom is sensitive to and respectful of the contributions the other can bring.

REFERENCES

Greenfield, S., Aronow, H.U., Elashoff, R.M., & Watanabe, D. (1988). Flaws in mortality data: The hazards of ignoring comorbid disease. *JAMA, 260*, 2,253–2,256.

Jencks, S.F., Daley, J., Draper, D., Thomas, D., Lenhart, G., & Walker, J. (1988). Interpreting hospital mortality data: The role of clinical risk adjustment. *JAMA, 260*, 3,611–3,616.

Kahn, K.L., Brook, R.H., Draper, D., Keeler, E.B., Rubenstein, L.V., Rogers, W.H., & Kosecoff, J. (1988). Interpreting hospital mortality data. How can we proceed? *JAMA, 260*, 3,625–3,628.

Kane, R.L., Lurie, N., Borbas, C., Morris, N., Flood, S., McLaughlin, B., Nemanich, G., & Schultz, A. (1995). The outcomes of elective laparoscopic and open cholecystectomies. *Journal of the American College of Surgeons, 180*(2), 136–145.

Radosevich, D.M., Kalambokidis, T.L., & Werni, A. (1996). *Practical guide for implementing, analyzing, and reporting outcomes measures.* Bloomington, MN: Health Outcomes Institute.

Spiegel, J.S., Ware, J.E., Ward, N.B., Kane, R.L., Spiegel, T.M., Paulus, H.E., & Leake, B. (1986). What are we measuring? An examination of self-reported functional status measures. *Arthritis and Rheumatism, 31*(6), 721–728.

NOTES

1. In many studies, the explained variance and regression coefficients do not precisely correspond to predictive variables because they describe associations that have been gathered retrospectively. They should be interpreted more cautiously. When a study uses what epidemiologists call a "case-control" model (i.e., it begins by identifying those with and without the outcome and looks for factors that are associated with one or the other), the best an investigator can do is to identify factors (i.e., treatments) that are likely to be more strongly associated with the outcome than its absence. These relationships are more appropriately expressed as *odds ratios*, which do not imply causal assumptions.

2. The term *risk factor* is used here in a generic sense to include all of the factors that can affect the outcomes of care. In some discussions of disease severity (see Chapter 6) *risk factor* is used interchangeably with *severity*. In this book, we have tried to use it consistently in the larger context.

3. For a practical guide to implementing quality improvement projects, see Radosevich, Kalambokidis, and Werni (1996).

Index _____

About the Author _____

Robert L. Kane, M.D., the editor of this book, holds an endowed chair in the University of Minnesota School of Public Health's Division of Health Services Research and Policy. He directs the University's Clinical Outcomes Research Center. Before accepting the endowed chair, he served as dean of the School of Public Health. He came to Minnesota after working as a Senior Researcher at the RAND Corporation and a professor at the UCLA Schools of Medicine and Public Health. Dr. Kane has been conducting studies on the outcomes of care for more than 20 years. His work, which has been supported by such organizations as the Agency for Health Care Policy and Research, the Health Care Financing Administration, the Robert Wood Johnson Foundation, the Pew Charitable Trusts, and the Commonwealth Foundation, has been directed at the outcomes of both ambulatory and institutional care. He is an active champion of using outcomes information to create financial incentives for better care. Because he views outcomes information as a dynamic enterprise that works best when information is collected prospectively, he prefers to think in terms of outcomes information systems rather than simply outcomes studies. He consults widely on the role of outcomes. He was a member of the Institute of Medicine committee on quality of care under Medicare.

The concept for this book grew out of a graduate seminar on outcomes research that was led by Dr. Kane. The contributors were all members of the seminar group. Their backgrounds are varied. Some are physicians with an interest in health services research; others are exclusively health services researchers. Although most chapters were individually authored, all members of the group played an active role in reviewing and modifying the work throughout its evolution.